Dr. Penny Stanway practised for several years as a GP and as a child-health doctor before becoming increasingly fascinated by researching and writing about a healthy diet and other natural approaches to health and wellbeing. She is an accomplished cook who loves eating and very much enjoys being creative in the kitchen and sharing food with others. Penny has written more than 20 books on health, food and the connections between the two. She lives with her husband in a houseboat on the Thames and often visits the south-west of Ireland. Her leisure pursuits include painting, swimming and being with her family and friends.

By the same author:

The Miracle of Lemons
The Miracle of Cider Vinegar
The Miracle of Bicarbonate of Soda (US – *The Miracle of Baking Soda*)
The Miracle of Olive Oil
The Miracle of Garlic
The Natural Guide to Women's Health
Healing Foods for Common Ailments
Good Food for Kids
Free Your Inner Artist
Breast is Best (revised and updated sixth edition, 2012)

As co-author:

Christmas – A Cook's Tour
The Lunchbox Book
Feeding Your Baby

THE MIRACLE OF
HONEY

Practical Tips for
HEALTH, HOME
& BEAUTY

DR. PENNY STANWAY

WATKINS PUBLISHING
LONDON

This edition first published in the UK and USA 2013 by
Watkins Publishing Limited
Sixth Floor, 75 Wells Street, London W1T 3QH

A member of Osprey Group

Design and typography copyright © Watkins Publishing Ltd. 2013

Text copyright © Dr Penny Stanway 2013

1 3 5 7 9 10 8 6 4 2

Designed and typeset by Jerry Goldie Graphic Design

Printed and bound in China

A CIP record for this book is available from the British Library

ISBN: 978-1-78028-500-9

www.watkinspublishing.co.uk

Distributed in the USA and Canada by Sterling Publishing Co., Inc.
387 Park Avenue South, New York, NY 10016-8810

For information about custom editions, special sales, premium and
corporate purchases, please contact Sterling Special Sales
Department at 800-805-5489 or specialsales@sterlingpub.com

Contents

DEDICATION

This book is dedicated to all those family members and friends who have joined me in the delightful pursuit of tasting honeys from around the world.

Introduction

Honey is a fragrant food made by honeybees. In ancient times, it was considered a food of the gods, a symbol of wealth, health and happiness and even an elixir of immortality. The Old Testament promised the Israelites 'a land flowing with milk and honey'. Egyptian doctors used honey-containing remedies 5,000 years ago. Mohammed claimed it was a remedy for every illness. And Hindus still use it today as one of the five foods offered in worship or welcome.

The word 'honey' comes from 'oneg', Hebrew for 'delight'. Honey is also known as the 'food of love'. Indeed, the word 'honeymoon' references the ancient Viking custom in which bride and groom consumed honey cakes and mead (a drink made by fermenting honey) for a month after betrothal. Today, bridegrooms in Morocco may follow tradition by feasting on honey.

A 100-million-year-old bee was recently found preserved in amber. We know people ate honey many thousands of years ago, but they have probably done so for much longer. They began by collecting honey from wild bees' nests, then progressed to keeping bees. Beekeeping was especially popular in Europe and so common in ancient Britain that it was called the 'land of honey'.

At first, honey was the only sweetener other than date, fig or maple syrup. Alexander the Great brought sugar cane from India to Greece in the 4th century bc. But only the rich could afford this 'honey reed' until the mass cultivation of sugar cane and sugar beet began in the

18th century. As sugar became more affordable, honey became less important.

The worldwide production of honey in 2010 was 1.4 million metric tons. China was the main honey-producer (22 per cent of global production), followed by the European Union (14 per cent), Argentina and the US (6 per cent each) and Turkey (5 per cent). Other honey producers, in order, are Ukraine, Mexico, the Russian Federation, Iran, Ethiopia, India, Tanzania, Spain, Canada, Kenya, Germany, Angola and Australia.

Honey consumption today is greatest in Greece at 1.62kg/3lb 5oz per person per year and lowest in Hungary at 0.18kg/6oz. In Canada, it is 0.78kg/1lb 11oz; Australia 0.6kg/1lb 4oz; the UK 0.59kg/1lb 5oz, the US 0.58kg/1.3lb and China 0.2kg/6oz.

In contrast, many consumers eat vastly more sugar. For example, the average person in the US consumes more than 70kg/156lb of sugar, including high-fructose corn syrup, each year – which is an awful lot of empty calories.

Neither the US nor most EU countries produce enough honey to meet their needs, so rely on imports. Britain produced only 15 per cent of its needs in 2009. And in 2010, Germany imported 80 per cent of the honey consumed there.

About 85 per cent of global production goes to consumers as table honey, the rest to the food industry for bakery, confectionery and breakfast cereals, for example. There is also a small market for honey in the pharmaceutical and tobacco industries.

The colour, consistency, fragrance and flavour of honey vary according to its nectar and honeydew sources as well as types of processing. Multifloral and blended honeys are most common, although consumers increasingly pay a premium for monofloral, raw or organic honey, and there is growing interest in darker, stronger-tasting honeys. Because just as wine or olive-oil aficionados delight in the differences between wines or oils from different seasons, producers and varieties of grape or olive, so too do honey lovers enjoy different honeys.

But not all is sweetness and light. Too many honeybees are dying, possibly because of pesticides, wildflower losses and bee malnutrition.

Hopefully, with care and research, our supplies of honey – and, most important, the pollination of food and other crops by honeybees – will become more secure and thus guarantee the survival of the honeybee.

CHAPTER ONE

Bees and Honey

Honeybees change nectar from flowers into honey, to make food for themselves. The average hive stores 9–14kg/20–30lb of honey by the end of the year. This represents a huge joint effort because a single worker bee produces only half a teaspoon of honey in her whole life. It takes nectar collections from around 2.6 million flowers, involving bee flights totalling around 88,000km/55,000 miles, to produce just 450g/1lb of honey.

The dates in this chapter are for temperate countries in the northern hemisphere. Adjust them by six months for temperate countries in the southern hemisphere.

Honeybees

Only a few of the 25,000 or so species of bee make honey, and most of these produce only tiny amounts.

Honeybees inhabit every continent except Antarctica. *Apis melllifera* is the most common type in Europe, the US, Canada and Australia. Honeybees live in large colonies and store a lot of honey. In contrast, the bumblebee (*Bombus bombus*) lives in a small colony that stores a tablespoon at most.

Honeybee varieties differ in honey-making ability, honeycomb colour and building, hive-care, immunity, tendency to swarm (form a new colony), multiplication, appetite and character. The most popular are Italians (brown-and-yellow-striped), Carniolans (black or grey) and Caucasians (grey). Thanks to migration and importation, though, many honeybees are mongrels today.

From here on I'll generally call honeybees simply 'bees'.

A bee colony

A bee colony – or family – consists of:

- A queen bee – the only fertile female. She lays eggs, keeps the colony happy, is the longest bee and lives 18 months on average, although she can survive up to six years.

- Up to 30,000-60,000 worker bees – small infertile females that groom and feed other bees, maintain the hive, collect nectar, pollen, propolis and water, and make honey. A spring- or summer-born worker lives six weeks at most, an autumn-born one six months.

- Several hundreds or thousands of drones – fertile males that are shorter and stouter than the queen, have large eyes but no sting, wax glands or pollen baskets, and live eight weeks at most.

The beehive

Wild bees build nests in trees, logs, hedges, cliffs or walls. Removing their honey destroys their nest. Over the centuries, people have designed reusable nests – 'hives' – that enable harvesting of honey without bothering the bees too much.

Worker bees fill the hive with vertical, double-sided sheets of wax honeycomb. Each side consists of hexagonal cells, most of which are 5–7mm/1.5–¼in across. These receive worker eggs and store the colony's food: honey, pollen and bee bread, a mixture of pollen, nectar, saliva and microorganisms. Slightly larger cells receive drone eggs, and very large, thimble-shaped ones receive queen eggs.

Many beekeepers supply honeycomb starter sheets so that bees don't need to make so much wax and, as a result, have more energy to make honey. These sheets encourage workers to build relatively few drone cells, whereas honeycomb built entirely by bees has more drone cells. This triggers the queen to lay more drone eggs, and it's said that having more drones makes a colony happier.

Honey is the bees' main source of carbohydrate, pollen their main source of protein. But both contain many other vital nutrients.

What each bee does

As a young adult, the queen couples with up to 40 drones. These then die, but she stores their semen. In April and May, the queen lays up to 3,000 eggs a day, each smaller than a grain of rice. Her fertilized eggs become workers and queens, while the unfertilized ones become drones.

After mating, and for the rest of her life, the queen's mandibular glands secrete a cocktail of 30 pheromones into her mouth. The scent of this 'queen substance' attracts workers to lick and feed her and to pass it on to other bees, which keeps them calm and cooperative.

The high-grade nourishment she needs comes from royal jelly, also called brood food or bee milk. This sweet, fatty, creamy-coloured substance contains whitish secretions from young workers' mandibular glands and yellowish protein-rich secretions from their hypopharyngeal glands.

Three days after being laid, the eggs hatch into larvae (grubs). These produce brood (or 'feed-me') pheromone whose scent stimulates workers to feed them. All larvae receive royal jelly at first.

Four days after hatching, workers choose a larva's food according to its cell size. Larvae in worker and drone cells stop receiving royal jelly and instead get bee bread, which is less nutritious. Larvae in queen cells continue to receive royal jelly – in fact, their cells are flooded with it – and this makes them develop into queens.

Six days after hatching, a larva spins a cocoon, and workers then seal its cell with a wax lid (capping), ready for pupation. During this stage, which lasts 10 days for a worker, 13 for a drone and five for a queen, a wondrous metamorphosis turns the larva into an adult bee. The young adult then chews through its cocoon and cell and emerges into the hive.

Worker bees

Up to 2,000 new young adult workers emerge each day from the average hive.

From one to seven days old, a worker is a 'nurse bee'. She cleans the hive. She solicits food by sticking out her proboscis ('tongue'), encouraging older bees to offer regurgitated honey. Later, she feeds herself from honey and bee-bread stores.

When pollen protein has matured her mandibular and hypopharyngeal glands, she feeds royal jelly to all young larvae and older queen larvae. She feeds older worker and drone larvae with bee bread. And she grooms and feeds young adults.

From 7–12 days, she is a 'house bee'. Her abdominal wax glands begin producing pinhead-sized scales of wax. Other bees collect her wax, soften it by chewing, then use it to build honeycomb and cap cells containing mature larvae or ripe honey. The latter is honey that has been dehydrated until its water content is about 20 per cent, so it resists fermentation. Once its cell is capped, its water content falls to about 18 per cent.

A house bee also strengthens, waterproofs and disinfects the hive, including the honeycomb, with propolis (see page 58).

From 12–14 days, a house bee converts nectar into honey. To do this, she accepts nectar from foragers, then for 30 minutes or so regurgitates a drop at a time, allowing invertase, an enzyme now produced by her hypopharyngeal glands, to break down sucrose into glucose and fructose. She holds each drop between her jaw and proboscis to encourage dehydration in the hive's warm air. She puts it down for several hours to allow further evaporation. Then she or another house bee puts it into a cell.

She also collects pollen pellets deposited by foragers, moistens them further with saliva and nectar, puts them into a cell and packs them down by head-butting. She covers pollen-filled cells with honey. Bacteria (lactobacilli) from secretions she has added to the honey ferment the pollen into bee bread. She also ejects debris from the hive.

From two weeks, a house bee dehydrates honey in uncapped cells by fanning her wings. And she guards the hive's entrance by sniffing other bees' scent. If it's foreign, she produces alarm pheromone to muster help.

At three weeks, she becomes a forager, flying out to collect nectar, pollen, propolis and water. She flies up to 1.6–3.2km/1–2 miles from the hive, sometimes three times as far, letting her scent receptors guide her to enticing scents, and her eyes to attractively coloured flowers. On a good dry day she might make 20 trips, each time visiting up to 1,000 flowers and sucking nectar through her proboscis and via her mouth into her honey sac (the expanded end of her gullet). She can feed on nectar by opening a valve in her honey sac to let some enter her stomach. She collects pollen by brushing it from her body with her middle legs, adding saliva and nectar to form tiny pellets, and packing these into hairy baskets on her back legs. She carries home 0.06g/0.002oz of nectar and

20mg/0.0007oz of pollen, equalling half her bodyweight. She collects water from ponds or other sources, or by choosing watery nectar, and carries it in her honey sac. She also collects propolis.

Once home, she lets other foragers smell and sample her nectar and pollen so they can decide whether to visit her sources. She regurgitates nectar for younger honeybees to ripen, and deposits pollen and propolis. She dances to alert other foragers to good nectar sources. A circle dance – first anti-clockwise, then clockwise – indicates nectar and/or pollen within 10m/11 yards. A waggle dance – half a circle one way, then a turn and a straight run while wagging her tail, then half a circle the other way – indicates they are more than 91m/100 yards away. The direction of the straight run indicates their location relative to the sun; the frequency of waggle runs defines their distance more precisely; her vigour communicates their quality.

Workers keep the hive at 28–35ºC/82.4–95ºF. They warm it by digesting honey and pollen, huddling together and shivering, and they cool it by distributing water and by fanning their wings near the entrance. They also wander around or rest, often breaking at midday when there is a lull in nectar production.

Foraging

Bees fly from the hive to collect nectars and pollens for food. Certain flower scents are especially attractive to foraging bees, and they particularly like blue and purple flowers. Indeed, a worker's two complex eyes, each with nearly 7,000 little lenses, are particularly sensitive to blue, purple and ultraviolet (UV) light. Nectar reflects UV light, and a worker detects this as a dark area in a flower. The other three of a worker's five eyes are simple eyes that sense polarized sunlight. Bees navigate by recognizing the landscape, and sensing the sun's position and the Earth's magnetic field.

A forager exhibits 'flower fidelity' by visiting only one type of flower per trip. Other bees in the colony may visit different types. Different nectars and pollens offer different proportions of their contents, encouraging a healthy diet.

Nectar

Nectar is a powerful attractant produced from sap by glands in a flower's nectaries. A hive's honey store is built up from many individual loads of nectar.

Honeybees have a short proboscis, so favour easily accessible nectar: for example, from flowers with a single ring of petals, multiple small flowers or a large trumpet.

Nectar is a watery solution of sugars, plus traces of acids, minerals, proteins, enzymes and various aromatic and other substances. Plants make sugars by photosynthesis. This involves converting water and carbon dioxide into oxygen and sugars using energy from light absorbed by the green plant pigment chlorophyll. Foragers prefer sweeter nectar because house-bees accept it more readily.

Nectar sugars vary in type and proportion according to a plant's species, and the soil, climate, weather and season. Sugars form 40-45 per cent of nectar by weight on average, but the proportion varies in different nectars. For example:

- Primrose   5
- Plum   15
- Apple   25
- Lime   35
- White clover   40
- Kale   50
- White horse-chestnut   70
- Marjoram   76

Nectar volume varies with flower species, soil moisture, air humidity and temperature, and rate of nectar flow. Nectar flow rises at certain times of day according to a flower's size and species. Temperature extremes can reduce or halt nectar production; warm weather increases it. Many wild flowers are excellent nectar producers.

This table (right) gives examples of the range of amounts of honey a colony of bees can make from 1 acre/2.5 hectares of land growing one type of plant:

Honeydew

Bees not only produce honey from nectar but also from honeydew, a sweet, dark or greenish liquid or crystalline substance excreted by aphids, leafhoppers and scale insects onto leaves or branches after eating sap. It's called honeydew because its droplets glisten like dew. Many honeys are made from both nectar *and* honeydew.

The manna referred to in the Bible was almost certainly honeydew.

Pollen

The nutrients in pollen include proteins (which strengthen bee-wing muscles), carbohydrate (which builds fat stores to provide energy for flying and warming the hive) and fats, vitamins, minerals and plant pigments (which promote general health).

Bees need pollens from a range of plants for optimal health. This is because the concentrations of nutrients vary in different plant species. Also, different plant pigments boost immunity in different ways.

Pollen can be yellow, orange, red, brown, black, green and even blue.

How much honey a bee colony makes per acre

PLANT	KG HONEY PER ACRE	LB HONEY PER ACRE
Tansy (phacelia)	82–682	180–1,500
Black locust	364–545	800–1,200
Lime	364–500	800–1,100
Rosebay willowherb (fireweed)	364	800
Coriander	91–159	200–350
Clover	91–136	200–300
Lemon balm (melissa)	68–114	150–250
Milkweed	54–114	120–250
Echium	91	200
Mint	68–91	150–200
Heather	45–91	100–200
Borage (starflower)	27–73	60–160
Cornflower	45–68	100–150
Thyme	23–68	50–150
Willow	45–68	100–150
Lavender	32–54	70–120
Hawthorn	23–45	50–100
Sunflower	14–45	30–100
Valerian	27–32	60–70
Elderberry	9–27	20–60
Goldenrod	11–23	25–50
Aster	14–23	30–50
Coltsfoot	11–16	25–35
Opium poppy	9–14	20–30

Season by season in a hive

A colony's activity varies with the seasons. The nearer the equator, the more even are the nectar and pollen supplies and therefore the honey production.

Spring

The only bees to survive winter are the queen and up to 10,000 workers. Hopefully, the colony has enough stored honey and pollen to feed them until enough early nectar and pollen is available. If not, the beekeeper can supply honey and pollen stored from the previous year in case of need.

Food supplements are second best. Patties of protein-rich substitute food made from soybean meal, milk, minerals, vitamins and high-fructose corn syrup are much better than sugar syrup. But even they are not nearly as nutritious as the bees' own honey and pollen.

Longer days, rising temperatures and good food supplies enable the queen to start laying, so plenty of workers will be available to collect nectar and pollen. Primed by good supplies of early nectar, the workers build honeycomb ready to store food for the growing brood. Supplies of protein from early pollens such as from coltsfoot and hazels are vital for healthy larvae.

Sources of nectar and pollen include certain trees (including willows and fruit trees), crops (such as avocado, borage, cotton, echium and winter-sown oilseed rape – canola), weeds (such as clover, coltsfoot and dandelion) and garden and wild plants (such as blackberry, crocuses, daffodils, elderberry, manuka, rosemary and tansy).

Most collected nectar and pollen feeds the growing colony. If nectar-flows are very good, though, beekeepers can harvest surplus honey. As spring-flower nectar and pollen supplies dwindle, some beekeepers move their hives to areas that will be rich in summer flowers.

By mid-May, egg-laying is at its height.

Summer

The average hive population peaks in mid-July, with up to 50,000 workers and up to 1,000 drones, plus a brood of 6,000 eggs, 9,000 larvae and 20,000 pupae. As brood-pheromone production by larvae is at its height, foragers have ample stimulation to collect food. Summer plants tend to have particularly sugary nectar that quickly builds honey stores. Sources include certain crops (such as blueberries, borage, buckwheat, lucerne – alfalfa, and spring-sown oilseed rape), weeds (such as dandelion, milkweed, purple loosestrife, rosebay willowherb or 'fireweed', sea lavender, smartweed, star-thistle, trefoil, and vetch) and garden and wild plants (such as aster, borage, goldenrod, heather, honeysuckle, lavender, melissa or 'lemon balm', sunflower and thyme).

Bees need plenty of nectar whose honey will remain runny for months in the comb and thus be easy to eat. Honey from certain nectars (such as aster, clover and oilseed rape) crystallizes within a few days and is difficult for bees to dilute and eat. If such nectars form the bulk of their spoils, bees may go hungry later in the year. Beekeepers harvest such honeys promptly so that they can remove it from the comb.

In some areas and in some seasons, late-summer nectar-producing flowers are scarce. Usually, though, a colony can store enough honey and pollen to sustain remaining bees through winter and get the new brood off to a good start in spring. If there is more than enough honey for the bees, beekeepers harvest some for themselves. If bees are making monofloral honey, beekeepers collect the surplus as soon as this nectar-flow ends. Beekeepers in Scotland, for example, may transport their bees to moorland in later summer to collect nectar from heather.

Autumn

The most northerly parts of temperate zones have few bee-friendly flowers from October to March. They include echium (second flowering), goldenrod, gorse (out for much of the year and visited mainly for pollen), heather and ivy. Falling temperatures make bees increasingly reluctant to forage, while shorter days reduce foraging time.

The queen lays fewer and fewer eggs. The last ones of the year become the workers that will raise the spring brood. To conserve food stores, workers kill remaining drones by starving them, pushing or excluding them from the hive or biting off their wings.

Some beekeepers wait until early September before removing their first honey of the year. Indeed, the US honey harvest traditionally begins on Labor Day (the first Monday in September). Two or more collections of surplus honey can usually be made each year, the last sometimes as late as in October, though some beekeepers make many more collections.

Winter

Short days prevent the queen laying eggs. The average colony shrinks to 10,000 bees at most. These stay active and eat the hive's food stores. If there isn't enough honey, or a beekeeper has taken too much, substitute food is vital or the colony will die.

If any nearby flowers blossom in January and the temperature is above 10ºC/ 50ºF, workers go out to forage.

If stored honey is very viscous, or has crystallized, bees dilute it with water before eating it.

Pollination

Pollination enables a plant to reproduce itself by producing seeds. It involves the transfer of pollen from the anthers (male organs) of one flower to the stigma (female organ) of another of the same species.

Flowers produce nectar to attract bees and other insects (and animals) to pollinate them. As a bee collects nectar, pollen collects on her hairy body. Her flower fidelity means she visits flowers of the same species and inadvertently pollinates them at the same time.

Most insect-pollinated flowers can be pollinated by a variety of insects. White clover, for example, is pollinated by honeybees, bumblebees and solitary bees. Others rely on only one sort of insect: for example, cocoa flowers are pollinated only by midges. Certain plants are pollinated by other animals (such as birds and bats); wind (for example, cereals, other grasses, most conifers and many deciduous trees); or humans (for example, greenhouse melons). And certain crops, including broad beans and coffee beans, can self-pollinate.

However, honeybees are the main pollinators of many plants, including many crops (such as almonds, apples, avocados, blueberries, cherries, cranberries, lettuce, oilseed rape and sunflowers). In 2011, a United Nations Environment Programme report noted that bees help pollinate more than 70 per cent of those 100 crops that supply 90 per cent of the world's food. In countries with a temperate climate, about a third of vegetable, fruit and nut crops, plus most wild flowers, depend on bee pollination.

A lack of bees limits the harvest from bee-pollinated crops. Some such crops, including almonds and blueberries, can crop without pollination, but this delays ripening; encourages damage by disease, poor weather, pests and pesticides; and produces fewer, smaller or seedless fruits.

All this has led to the vast industry of migratory beekeeping. Farmers pay beekeepers to transport bees sometimes thousands of miles to pollinate crops such as almonds, apples, blueberries, borage, field beans and oilseed rape. In the US, more than 2.5 million hives are rented to farms each year. One million, for example, go to almond orchards in California; 50,000 to blueberry fields in Maine; and 30,000 to apple orchards in New York State.

Challenges to bees ... and humans

In recent years, bee numbers have declined steeply. Around a third of the bee population was lost in the US in 2007–2008. The number of bees in the UK has halved from the 1960s to 2012. Large losses have been reported in Egypt, China and Japan.

This is alarming because a third of our food comes from crops that rely mainly on bees to pollinate them. A lack of bees not only makes harvests small, unreliable and late, but wildflowers dwindle because there are so few seeds, and there is less honey for bees – and humans – to eat.

The death of the queen bee is associated with one in four colony losses, while 'colony-collapse disorder' in which a whole bee colony goes missing, presumed dead, accounts for about 7 per cent of losses in the US, rather fewer in Europe.

The subject of colony collapse is much debated and theories abound as to the cause. One suggestion is that lead-containing crystals in bees' abdomens sensitize them to the growing number of electromagnetic fields surrounding us, influencing their behaviour and encouraging disease. Another is that infestation with *Varroa destructor* mites, or infection with viruses, fungi or bacteria, makes bees more vulnerable to disease. Yet another is that vehicle-exhaust fumes react with airborne scent molecules from flowers, making them confusing and unattractive to bees.

But the three most important reasons for the declining number of bees seem to be malnutrition, insecticides and stress. Because these are so important for the future of worldwide honey production, we'll look at each in detail.

Bee malnutrition

A main cause is **shrinkage of wildflower habitats** reducing the volume and variety of nectars and pollens. In the UK, for example, wildflower populations have fallen by 95 per cent since the destruction of hedgerows accompanying the need for food production after World War 2. Weedkillers and single-crop farming are also to blame. Worryingly, one in five species of wildflower risks extinction.

The other main cause is the **poor nutritional quality of food substitutes** such as sugar syrup given to bees if honey stores are low or beekeepers have harvested too much. Malnourished bees are more vulnerable to insecticides, infections and parasites.

A colony needs only 9–14kg/20–30lb of honey to survive the average winter, but can store much more given enough space and successful foraging. In an average year, the average colony in a UK Modified National Hive produces a surplus of 10–14kg/22–30lb. In a good season, a strong colony can produce an extra 18–27kg/40–60lb. And some colonies produce an extra 36–45kg /80–100lb or more. One Australian beekeeper took 285kg/629lb per hive when the flow of eucalyptus nectar was particularly good.

Good beekeepers remove only the honey likely to be surplus to the bees' needs. Others take as much as possible and give the bees substitute food. The best substitutes contain protein, carbohydrate, fat, vitamins and minerals. But even these are limited in their range and quality of nutrients and other phytochemicals compared with pollen and honey. The poorest substitute, sugar syrup, provides vastly less nourishment.

However, it must be said that if bees can't make enough honey for their needs, or if honey sets so firmly in the comb that they can't eat it, substitute food given by beekeepers can save their lives.

Exposure of bees to insecticides

At worst, certain insecticides used on farms, gardens, recreational areas, parks, forests, marshes, swamps and hives kill bees outright. Repeated low doses weaken their resistance to infection.

Stress on bees

Bees can become stressed by poorly designed hives, overly frequent inspections and lengthy travel when migratory beekeepers take them to pollinate and produce honey from far-away crops.

The future

The way things are going, there will be fewer and fewer bees, less and less honey and a crash in bee-pollinated crop production. But with individual and communal action we can prevent this horrendous scenario.

Give wildflowers a chance

We can encourage wildflowers by sowing them in gardens, parks, on banks and verges, and around crop-bearing fields. Mowing several times in the first year discourages perennial weeds from taking over. A well-chosen mixture of species can prolong flowering by 6–8 weeks and provide more food for bees.

Farmers can sow bee-friendly wildflowers such as wild carrot that flower after a main crop such as wheat and, as an added bonus, reduce the need for weedkillers. They can also cut hay late to give wild flowers more chance to bloom. State-funded set-aside schemes are good since unploughed farmland encourages wildflowers.

Favour bee-friendly ornamental flowers

Gardens, parks and other display areas can be planted with bee-friendly flowers. These include alyssum, asters, borage, candytuft, catmint, coreopsis, daffodils, single dahlias, echium, French marigolds, goldenrod, heather, honeysuckle, larkspur, lavender, lemon balm, nasturtium, rosemary, scabious, sea holly, sedum, sunflowers, sweet william, thyme and tobacco plants.

Bee-friendly flowers are preferable to ones that are showy but offer little nectar (such as begonias, busy lizzies, double dahlias and bedding geraniums). Note that bees favour flowers in clumps and sunny places.

Use insecticides with care, if at all

Instructions should be followed precisely, with applications timed so levels are low during flowering; open flowers should never be sprayed; and spraying should be done only in the evenings or on dull days when fewer bees are about. Good communication between farmers and beekeepers enables hives to be moved before crops are sprayed.

Insecticidal seed dressings called neonicotinoids are of greatest concern. As a seed develops into a plant, they spread through the whole plant and into its nectar and pollen.

Repeated low-level exposure seems to damage bees' navigational skills and memory. They may then lose their way to the hive and die. Studies in France, Scotland and the UK have linked neonicotinoids with bee deaths. Researchers at Royal Holloway College in London, for example, studied nearly 1,000 bees from 40 colonies throughout the UK. Each was tagged with a microchip and some were given a cocktail of pesticides mimicking those commonly encountered on crops. After release, those given pesticides were much less likely to return.

However, one major manufacturer says that neonicotinoids are safe for bees and withdrawing them does not improve bee health.

The dilemma for national regulators is that without pesticides we might lose 30 per cent of our crops. But with them, an ongoing decline in bee numbers could give the same result. A great many people would favour bees rather than pesticides. But big business has a lot of clout.

Honey production is under threat in many countries, but we know some of the ways in which we can help. We just need to act.

CHAPTER TWO

What's in Honey

Honey is a wonderfully complex and exotic food. Each honey is a unique blend of 200 or so constituents that vary with its nectar and honeydew sources. Honey also contains tiny amounts of pollen, bee enzymes and microorganisms, and fragments of beeswax and propolis (see page 58).

Sugars form around 81 per cent of honey's weight. Next is water, at 14–18 per cent. The remaining three per cent include enzymes, acids, proteins, plant pigments, minerals, vitamins and various other substances. One tablespoon of honey supplies about 22 calories of energy and 17g of carbohydrate as sugars.

Sugars

Honey contains 24 different sugars. In contrast, 'table' sugar contains only one: namely, sucrose. The proportions of sugars vary in different honeys. The particular cocktail of sugars in any one honey contributes to its flavour and health benefits.

Glucose (formerly called 'dextrose') and fructose ('levulose') form about 73 per cent of honey's weight. The proportions of these simple sugars (monosaccharides) are roughly equal, although they vary with a honey's nectar and honeydew sources, so some honeys have relatively more fructose than glucose, and vice versa. Fructose is sweeter, so fructose-rich honeys are particularly sweet. The more glucose in a honey, the faster it crystallizes and thickens.

Much less important by weight are certain disaccharides whose molecules are each made of two linked simple sugars. They include sucrose, at about 1 per cent, and maltose and many others (such as gentiobiose, isomaltulose, kojibiose, lactose, maltulose, melibiose, nigerose, trehalose and turanose) at about 7 per cent.

Last are certain other monosaccharides (such as arabinose, galactose and mannose); trisaccharides (including centose, dextrantriose, kestose, maltotriose, panose and theanderose); tetrasaccharides (such as stachyose); and some more complex sugars, including isomaltotetraose.

Sugars whose molecules are each made of from two to nine linked simple sugars are also called oligosaccharides. Some, including kojibiose, maltose, nigerose and turanose, have particular health benefits.

Honeydew-containing honeys contain less fructose, glucose and sucrose, but more maltose and certain other oligosaccharides. Certain sugars, including the trisaccharides erlose, melezitose and raffinose, are present only in honeydew-containing honeys. Melezitose makes honey crystallize rapidly. If it forms 20 per cent by weight or more, the honey thickens so much that it hardens into 'cement honey'.

Certain sugars are produced by enzymes during the bees' production of honey; others by chemical changes during storage.

Health benefits
Honey's sugars are all converted to glucose in our body and are responsible for almost all the energy it provides. They also have other positive health effects.

Glucose – can release hydrogen peroxide, which is an antimicrobial and, perhaps, an anti-cancer agent.

Oligosaccharides – are prebiotics, meaning they aid the growth and activity of 'good' (probiotic) gut bacteria such as lactobacilli and bifido-bacteria and suppress those of harmful ones by stopping them sticking to the bowel wall. Probiotic bacteria aid digestion and may discourage certain gastrointestinal disorders, including colon cancer, diarrhoea and irritable bowel. Their presence in traces of honey in the mouth and throat helps prevent upper respiratory infections by discouraging bacteria such as pneumococci and *Haemophilus influenzae* from adhering to the mucous membrane. There's also some evidence that they help prevent flu, urine infection, high blood pressure, inflammation, high cholesterol and poor immunity.

Adding honey to yogurt or other fermented dairy products feeds their probiotic bacteria, boosting their growth and activity.

Certain honeys are particularly rich in oligosaccharides. Some (such as New Zealand Honeyco's Beech Forest Honeydew) are given a bioactivity rating according to their oligosaccharide content: 10+ is high, 20+ very high. Most honeys would score only 3+.

Water

Honey's usual water content of 16–18 per cent prevents wild yeasts multiplying. Any more watery and honey is likely to ferment. The water content of raw honey can be as low as 14 per cent.

Enzymes

As bees convert nectar into honey, their hypopharyngeal glands release enzymes, including:

- Invertase, which converts nectar's sucrose into glucose and fructose. (The digestive enzyme sucrase does the same in our body, but in a different way.)

- Amylases, which break down starch and include diastase
  (see page 35).

- Glucose oxidase, which converts glucose into gluconic acid and
  hydrogen peroxide (as in hair bleach) when honey is diluted with
  water and its acidity falls, and when there is sufficient sodium.

- Others, including catalase and inulase.

Darker honeys contain higher levels of enzymes. Enzymes are inactivated
by bright light and excessive heat, which is partly why a beehive's interior
is very dark and its temperature is regulated by worker bees.

Health benefits

Honey's enzymes remain at full strength if a honey is never heated beyond
40°C/104°F.

Invertase – by 'predigesting' some of nectar's sucrose, this enables
someone who lacks sucrase (for example, because of gastroenteritis) to
eat honey without getting diarrhoea from undigested sucrose passing
through the bowel.

Glucose oxidase – is released from honey's glucose in the presence
of water, which reduces acidity, and sodium from food, drink, gastric
or intestinal juice, or wound fluid. It facilitates hydrogen-peroxide
production.

Acids

Honey is moderately acidic, thanks mostly to its many organic acids.
The main one is gluconic acid. Others include acetic, citric, forminic,
malic and succinic acids and phenolic acids such as caffeic, cinnamic and

ferrulic acids. Honey also contains tiny amounts of fatty acids and about 18 amino acids, including lysine, proline and tryptophan.

Honey's acidity is indicated by its pH (potential of Hydrogen: where pH 0–7 is acidic, 7 neutral and 7–14 alkaline). The pH of different honeys ranges from 3.2–4.5. Honey's acidity is similar to that of orange juice.

The amounts and types of acids vary with a honey's nectar and honeydew sources. Darker honeys are usually more acidic. Storing honey slightly increases its acidity. Honey's acidity makes it resistant to fermentation, one of the reasons why it keeps so well.

Health benefits
Honey's acidity is antibacterial.

Raw honey's acidity makes it an alkali-producing food. A typical westernized diet has an acid-producing effect that causes chronic metabolic low-grade 'acidosis'. In this condition, the blood is slightly less alkaline than ideal, which is thought to trigger many health problems.

In contrast, processed honey produces acid – and sugar is an even more acid-producing food.

Vitamins and minerals

Honey contains small amounts of vitamins A, B, including folic acid, C, D, E and K. The vitamin C content of different honeys varies from 5–150mg per 100g, depending mainly on how much pollen there is in a honey.

Honey also has small amounts of minerals, including aluminium, calcium, chromium, chlorine, copper, iron, magnesium, manganese, phosphorus, potassium, selenium, silica, sodium, sulphur and zinc. The amounts depend on the mineral content of the soil that nurtured the plants from which a honey's nectar and honeydew sources originated. Darker honeys are usually richer in minerals.

Health benefits

The amounts of honey's vitamins and minerals are small, but help meet our needs.

Consuming 1.2g of honey per 1kg bodyweight nearly doubles the blood's vitamin C.

Polyphenols

Derived from phenolic acid and also called phenolic compounds, their amounts vary with the levels in their floral sources. Many are antioxidants, and some are phytoestrogens. The main honey polyphenols are flavonoids (see below); others include caffeic, protochatechuic, vanillic and gallic acids.

Health benefits

Honey's polyphenols are antioxidants (see 'Antioxidants', pages 24–5), some being more effective than vitamin C.

Early evidence suggests certain non-flavonoid polyphenols are phytoestrogens (plant oestrogens) that can have oestrogenic effects in the human body by attaching to and activating oestrogen receptors on cells.

Studies of phytoestrogens in other foods show they affect people differently:

- In a woman with high levels of her own oestrogens, phytoestrogens attaching and activating her cells' oestrogen receptors prevent her oestrogens attaching. Because activation by her oestrogens would have had stronger effects, the attachment of phytoestrogens decreases her body's oestrogenic activity. This could be useful if she has an oestrogen-dominant hormone imbalance causing, for example, bloating, cyclical weight gain, endometriosis, fibroids, heavy or irregular periods, infertility, irritability, lumpy tender breasts, miscarriage, nausea, polycystic ovary syndrome, postmenopausal bleeding, thickened womb lining, vaginal discharge or womb, ovary or breast cancer.

- In a woman with low levels of her own oestrogens (for example, after the menopause), phytoestrogens attaching and activating her cells' oestrogen receptors increase her body's oestrogenic activity. This could be useful if she has an oestrogen deficiency causing, for example, acne, depression, dry vagina, fatigue, greasy hair and skin, infertility, irregular periods, low sex drive, non-cyclical weight gain or abnormal hairiness.

Very little research has examined the effects of phytoestrogens in men.

Flavonoids

These plant pigments have been called bioflavonoids and vitamin P. They include acacetin, apigenin, biochanin, chrysin, eriodictyol, formonontin, galangin, genistein, hesperetin, kaempferol, liquiriteginin, luteolin, myricetin, naringenin, pinobanksin, pinocembrin, pinostrobin and quercetin.

Health benefits

Honey's flavonoids are antioxidant (see below), anti-microbial, anti-allergic and anti-inflammatory. They improve vitamin C absorption, protect collagen, our most abundant protein, and aid cell communication ('cell-signalling'). This latter property helps cells work properly.

Honey's flavonoids may also have anti-cancer effects.

Antioxidants

Honey's main antioxidants are flavonoids. Others include other polyphenols, enzymes, organic acids, other plant pigments, peptides (protein fragments) and terpenes, as well as salicylic acid (aspirin), vitamins C and E, selenium and zinc. Their combined effect is much greater than expected from their individual amounts.

Certain honeys have an antioxidant level 150 times higher than others. The level varies according to the amounts and types of the nectar and honeydew sources.

Health benefits

Honey's antioxidants discourage the oxidation of cholesterol and other fats that increases when the body is stressed by, for example, smoking, too much sun or exercise, or an unhealthy diet, and can cause inflammation and cell damage.

Certain honeys are particularly rich in antioxidants. Others are allocated a bioactivity rating according to their antioxidant content: 10+, for example, is high and 20+ very high. In contrast, clover honey only scores 3+. In contrast, an apple would score 4+, broccoli 10+, blueberries 19+, spinach 20+ and blackcurrants 32+.

Antimicrobials

Some honeys are 100 times more powerfully antimicrobial than others. The possible antimicrobials include:

- Hydrogen peroxide, produced if added water activates the enzyme glucose oxidase. It accounts for most of the antibacterial activity of most honeys.

- Flavonoids in particular as well as pinocembrin.

- Phenolic acids such as caffeic and ferulic acids.

- Methylglyoxal, present in certain manuka and jellybush honeys in levels up to 1,000 times higher than in other honeys, and doubled in antibacterial activity by an unknown synergist in these honeys.

- Sugars.

- Furanones.

- Defensin-1, apidaecins and abaecin, which are proteins that bees add to honey.

Methylglyoxal – a byproduct of sugar metabolism that is present in many foods and drinks and is also produced by gut bacteria. Methylglyoxal in manuka honey is dubbed 'unique manuka factor' (UMF). In jellybush honey it's called 'unique leptospermum factor' (ULF) as 'UMF' is trade-marked. Some jellybush honeys contain more methylglyoxal than the richest manuka honeys.

Medical-grade honey – is heated only minimally, then passed through a fine filter and gamma-irradiated to kill microorganisms. It's checked for pesticide residues and heavy metals and sold in dark-glass containers so that light cannot destroy its antimicrobials. Some honeys, including certain manuka honeys, are produced as medical-grade. Medical-grade honey is also used to make certain medical honey-containing products such as honey-impregnated wound dressings.

Health benefits

Honey's antimicrobials inactivate or kill more than 250 strains of bacteria and certain fungi, including *Candida albicans* and viruses. Honey's anti-infective power depends on its nectar and honeydew sources and its processing.

Because honey contains hundreds of antibacterial compounds, bacteria are highly unlikely to become resistant. The compounds are quickly absorbed into the blood, so don't destroy 'good' bowel bacteria.

Hydrogen peroxide – is effective even though present in a 1,000-fold smaller amount than in a typical hydrogen-peroxide wound disinfectant. It has a valuable slow-release action. It also stimulates white cells that boost immunity.

Furanones – act against biofilms, slimy sheets of bacteria that are much more resistant to antibiotics and antiseptics than free bacteria.

Methylglyoxal – Certain honeys have a bioactivity rating according to the antibacterial strength of their methylglyoxal. Manuka honey can have a UMF (unique manuka factor) rating, and jellybush honey a ULF (unique leptospermum factor) rating. A rating of 5, for example, means it's as strong as a 5 per cent solution of phenol, an antiseptic. A rating of 0–4 indicates undetectable methylglyoxal; 5–9, low levels; 10–15, therapeutically useful levels; and 16–30, high potency.

Manuka honey with a UMF or ULF of 10 or more can act against biofilms and skin infections with antibiotic-resistant bacteria such as MRSA (methicillin-resistant *Staphylococcus aureus*). It doesn't have this action in blood.

The term 'Active Manuka Honey' was coined for manuka honeys with antibacterial activity from methylglyoxal rather than hydrogen peroxide. But some honeys are now labelled 'Active Manuka Honey' even though their antibacterial activity results mainly, as in most honeys, from their hydrogen peroxide.

In the test tube, methylglyoxal can damage genes and cells. Large amounts have been linked with premature ageing, cancer and reduced efficacy of insulin, the hormone that lets blood glucose enter cells.

Methylglyoxal is safe for healthy people as their cells break down much of it. But this may not happen in people with diabetes, so researchers are concerned it may then do damage by attaching to certain body proteins. Damage to insulin could worsen diabetes, while damage to certain other proteins could encourage Alzheimer's and Parkinson's.

Until we know more, it's probably better for people with diabetes and, perhaps, pre-diabetes too to avoid consuming manuka or jellybush honey. Interestingly, the diabetes drug metformin was designed to reduce methyl-glyoxal's insulin-damaging effects.

Sugars – attract water, thus dehydrating and deactivating local bacteria and fungi.

'Good' bacteria

Honey can also contain probiotic lactobacilli and bifidobacteria that discourage the overgrowth of potentially harmful gut bacteria.

These gut-friendly bacteria come from bees' honey sacs and are generally present only in honey less than two to three months old. Summer honey has the highest levels.

They are absent in honey from bees fed with sugar supplements.

Health benefits

Honey's 'good' bacteria increase the proportion of probiotic bowel bacteria (see page 20).

Immunity boosters

These include hydrogen peroxide (see page 27) and the protein 5.8-kDa.

Health benefits

Honey stimulates immune cells to produce anti-inflammatory cytokines such as interleukin-1 and -6 and tumour necrosis factor, which can destroy certain cancer cells.

Bitters

Certain honeys contain very small amounts of bitter substances ('bitters') from various nectars or honeydews, including almond, chestnut, goldenrod, hawthorn, ivy, manuka, onion, pine, privet, ragwort, sourwood, strawberry tree, tree of heaven, wild parsley and yew. They include certain glycosides, alkaloids, polyphenols and terpenoids.

Bees avoid very bitter nectars and honeydews, but collect slightly bitter ones and are particularly attracted to those containing nicotine or caffeine.

Many people enjoy slight bitterness; others dislike it; and some are genetically unable to taste it. A very few honeys are unacceptably bitter. Processors can reduce bitterness by blending in other honeys.

The following bitters can enhance a honey's flavour:

- Amygdalin – from almond trees

- Caffeine – from citrus (especially grapefruit) and coffee trees

- Capsaicin – from chili plants

- Cocaine – from coca bushes

- Codeine, heroin, morphine and opium – from opium poppies

- Convallotoxin – from lilies of the valley

- Gossypol – from cotton plants

- Hederagenin – from ivy

- Nicotine – from tobacco

- Tannins – from oak trees

- Tetrahydrocannabinols – from marijuana plants

If present in sufficient amounts, and if enough honey is consumed, very few bitters can cause symptoms or even threaten life. They include:

- Aconitine – from aconite

- Aesculin – from horse-chestnut trees

- Atropine, hyoscyamine and scopolamine – from deadly nightshade (*Atropa belladonna*), datura and henbane (stinking nightshade; *Hyoscyamus niger*). Small quantities of datura honey can cause inebriation.

- Gelsemine – from yellow jasmine.

- Granayotoxin – from bog rosemary (*Andromeda polifolia*), *Kalmia* species such as sheep laurel and mountain laurel (calico bush or spoon-wood), pieris and *Rhododendron ponticum* (also called *Azalea ponticum*). This can cause 'honey intoxication', with sweating, nausea, vomiting, diarrhoea, fainting, dizziness, breathing problems, weakness, irregular heartbeat and convulsions. These symptoms usually last less than a day and are rarely fatal. But eating as much as 14 tablespoons of mountain laurel honey, for example, could kill a 68kg/150lb person.

- Oleandrin – from oleander

- Pyrrolizidine alkaloids – see below

- Swainsonine – from spotted locoweed (*Astragalus lentiginosus*)

- Tutin – from tutu (*Coriaria arborea*)

- Unknown substances in the wharangi bush (*Melicope ternate*)

Pyrrolizidine alkaloids(PAs) are present in 3 per cent of plants. They number more than 660 and include lasiocarpine in comfrey; lycopsamine in borage; and jacoline and jacozine in ragwort. Most PA-containing plants belong to the asteraceae (including ragwort and groundsel), boraginaceae (including comfrey and echiums) and leguminosae (including peas, beans and rattleworts) families. Ragwort is the most common.

Various foods, including milk, grains, eggs and honey, can contain PAs. Particularly if eaten frequently and in large amounts, one in two PAs can encourage liver disease and cancer, and damage unborn babies. However, reports of poisoning are rare, and most result from herbal remedies or teas. At the time of writing, there is no international regulation of PA levels in foods unlike for herbal remedies.

Any risk from PAs in honey is unclear, but there is probably no problem because their bitterness makes nectar less attractive to bees. Also, any PA would be present in only a very small amount after dilution in the hive by nectar and honeydew from other sources. Finally, processors tend to blend bitter honey with other honeys, which dilutes any PAs that are present. Lastly, beekeepers try to site their hives to minimize any risk from PAs.

Health benefits
Honey's bitters stimulate bile flow, which aids digestion and discourages gallstones.

Acetylcholine and choline

Honey contains small amounts of these. They are also produced in our body.

Health benefits
Honey's acetylcholine can boost a low level of our own acetylcholine, a neurotransmitter or nerve-message carrier. Its effects include slowing the heartbeat, encouraging stomach and bowel movements, improving

memory and concentration, and widening blood vessels.

Honey's choline can contribute to our body's requirement for this essential nutrient. Choline is particularly important to our brain, heart, liver, muscle and cell membranes, and in pregnancy.

Scent and flavour compounds

Each honey has a unique aroma and taste. Experienced 'noses' and tasters identify the flavours in honeys as being floral, aromatic-herbal, fresh, citric, fresh-fruit, ripe-fruit, caramel, woody or hay-like.

More than 500 volatile compounds, many from essential oils in nectar, contribute to honey's scent and flavour. Many are aldehydes and ketones; others are acids such as cinnamic acid (which smells of honey) alcohols, bitters, esters and terpenes. There may also be aromatic alcanes from beeswax. Non-volatile compounds such as sugars, flavonoids and amino acids also contribute to honey's flavour.

A unique cocktail of up to 60 compounds accounts for the scent of each plant's essential oil, with larger amounts of several compounds characterizing each cocktail. This is why, for example, derivatives of the aldehyde linalool (with its floral, slightly spicy smell) characterize citrus honeys; dihydroxyketones characterize eucalyptus honeys; and the aldehydes hexanal (with its scent of freshly mown grass) and heptanal (fresh, herbal, green, woody, fruity) characterize lavender honeys.

Prolonged heating at more than 35°C/95°F changes a honey's scent and flavour by evaporating volatile aromatic compounds and beginning to burn its sugars.

Health benefits

Honey's volatile aromatic molecules stimulate sensory nerve endings in the nose. Enjoying the scent can lift the spirits. What's more, certain molecules have relaxing or stimulating effects in the brain.

Certain aromatic compounds absorbed into the blood (via the lining of the nose or breathing passages; or from honey on the skin or in the stomach or gut) can affect health. Linalool, for example, can have sedative effects.

Other substances

These include pollen, rich in vitamin C and protein, small amounts of bees' salivary enzymes, plant-growth hormones, rooting compounds and fragments of beeswax, propolis and bees' body parts.

Honey also contains tiny amounts of lipids from plants' essential oils. They include certain fatty acids (such as palmitic, oleic acid, lauric, stearic and linoleic acids), hydrocarbons, waxes, cholesterol esters, fatty-acid esters, fatty alcohols, sterols, di- and trihydroxy compounds, and polyol esters. Some contribute to honey's scent and flavour.

Adulterants

These can be added by beekeepers, processors or packers. The possibilities include:

- Sugars and other carbohydrates (for example, high-fructose corn syrup, invert-sugar syrup, glucose, molasses, flour and starch).

- Water.

- Environmental contaminants such as pesticides and lead (for example, from vehicle-exhaust fumes).

- Bee and hive medications (such as antibiotics and fungicides).

- Chemicals from plastic (if honey has been heated in plastic pots).

Legal standards for honey quality and tests for adulteration vary from country to country. However, the Codex Alimentarius, compiled by the United Nations Food and Agriculture Organization, requires there to be no adulteration with sugar or water of honey sold to the public.

Batches of honey can be tested for hydroxymethylfurfural (HMF), produced when simple sugars, especially fructose, break down in acidic conditions. A high level may indicate adulteration with sugar syrup, over-heating or lengthy storage. Hot climates can raise HMF to over 100mg/kg. Certain countries require a limit of 100mg/kg in imported honey. Bulk-traded honey must usually have an HMF below 10–15mg/kg so as to enable further processing and a longer shelf life before the 40 mg/kg level is reached.

Invert-sugar syrup (including high-fructose corn syrup)

This contains fructose, glucose and, for high-fructose corn syrup, a little maltose. It's cheap to make, so adding it to honey increases profits. This is most likely in the production of cheap imported blended honeys. Indeed, in certain countries syrup-adulterated, or 'stretched', honey is widely available. Astonishingly, stretched honeys containing up to 80 per cent corn syrup are sometimes labelled 'pure honey'! This dupes consumers into buying what they think is honey, but is actually sugar syrup plus honey.

In 2009, the state of Florida prohibited the addition of adulterants such as sugar syrup to products labelled 'honey'. The US now needs a similar federal law. Strict labelling regulations are required in certain other countries, too.

High-fructose corn syrup (HFCS) is produced by milling corn, processing the resulting corn starch to yield corn syrup, which is almost entirely glucose, then adding enzymes to convert some of this glucose into fructose. The most common, HFCS 55, contains 55g of fructose,

41g of glucose and 4g of maltose per 100g and is 25 per cent sweeter than sugar. Next most common is HFCS 42, with 42g of fructose, 53g of glucose and 5g of maltose and roughly as sweet as sugar.

Another sort of invert-sugar syrup is produced by heating sucrose from sugar cane or beet with acid, or adding invertase, to convert it into glucose and fructose.

Testing for HMF (see page 34) indicates whether a honey is likely to have been adulterated with syrup.

Officials can also test by measuring the activity of the enzyme diastase. This also indicates quality because activity is low if a honey has been:

- Adulterated with syrup (as this dilutes diastase).

- Damaged by overheating (as this destroys diastase).

- Stored a long time (as this gradually reduces diastase).

Some honey adulterers, though, disguise the fall in diastase by adding foreign diastase.

Antibiotics, fungicides and mite-killing medications

Beekeepers use medications to prevent or treat infestation of bees with Varroa mites or to treat bacterial or fungal disease. Various measures can minimize the amounts entering honey.

Interestingly, as mites dislike the scent of certain essential oils, they are less likely to infest a hive if its honey and propolis originate from plants producing these oils. Such plants include coriander and lavender, so it's worth planting these near hives.

Ongoing concern about honey from China dates from certain of their beekeepers using the antibiotic chloramphenicol to treat an epidemic of the bee disease foulbrood that began in 1997. They then exported chloramphenicol-contaminated honey. This antibiotic is toxic to humans, causing a potentially fatal disease called aplastic anaemia in a few of those exposed to even small amounts. Other potentially dangerous antibiotics, including ciprofloxacin, have also been found in Chinese honey.

Regulations were tightened following the scandal over imports of contaminated honey into the EU (European Union) and US. The EU, for example, now requires imported honey to be free from prohibited residues such as certain antibiotics, pesticides and heavy metals.

However, officials suspect very large amounts of honey continue to enter from China into the EU and the US via countries such as India and Vietnam. One reason for this suspected 'honey laundering' is that countries such as India export vastly more honey than they could possibly produce.

In 2008, the US imposed steep anti-dumping trade tariffs on Chinese honey, and its Customs Border Protection stepped up testing of imported honey. The EU has prohibited imports of honey from non-EU countries that are not on the 'Third Country Listing'. Countries on this list must test samples of honey destined for export. In 2010, the EU banned honey from India because there was insufficient clarity about its origin and possible adulteration with invert-sugar syrup or contamination with antibiotics and heavy metals.

Ever-improving measures are vital to prevent fraud.

Pesticides

Bees can make contaminated honey if pesticides have been sprayed on open flowers or systemic pesticides have been applied to a crop. Systemic pesticides spread into nectar. Consuming contaminated nectar can damage bee health. And consuming contaminated honey could, at worst, and if done regularly, damage human health.

Several measures can prevent or reduce pesticide contamination (see page 17).

CHAPTER THREE

Choosing and Using Honey

Honeys vary in colour, thickness, clarity, scent and flavour depending on their nectar and honeydew sources, their processing and their storage.

Honey products

Honey is arguably best eaten **warm from the hive**. Most of us, though, purchase honey from grocery stores, supermarkets, farmers' markets or even online.

Honeycomb 'sections' are sold in small wooden frames taken from a hive's honey boxes ('supers'). Pieces of honeycomb packed in wooden or plastic containers are called **cut-comb honey**. **Chunk honey** comes as a jar of runny honey containing one or more pieces of honeycomb. When eating honeycomb, some people chew it like gum, then either swallow the bits of wax or spit them out. Honeycomb is easier to eat if beekeepers have furnished hives with commercially made beeswax starter sheets. This is because their wax is thinner than in honeycomb made entirely by bees.

Most honey comes as **runny** or **thick honey**. Both have been drained or pressed from the comb, or spun out by a rotary extractor. Thick honey has either crystallized (granulated) and therefore thickened naturally or has been 'creamed' (see page 40). Runny honey is sometimes presented in squeezy plastic bottles rather than glass or ceramic jars or pots. It's also sold in sealed single-use plastic straws (honey sticks) so that it can easily be added to coffee or ice cream, for example, away from home.

Heating

After being extracted from the comb, most honey is heated to:

- Reduce its viscosity, to ease straining (or filtering) and bottling (packing).

- Delay crystallization, to keep it runny for longer.

- Kill yeasts, to prevent fermentation.

Heat of more than 40ºC/104°F begins to evaporate honey's volatile flavour compounds and inactivate its enzymes, while more than 49ºC/120ºF destroys the enzymes.

However, most commercially available honeys are heated to 66ºC/150ºF (pasteurized) to deter crystallization and fermentation. Heating to this temperature or higher also enables a process called ultra-filtration, in which honey is pressurized through a very fine filter to make it very clear and remaining runny for longer. The faster honey is heated and subsequently cooled, the less damage there is.

Colour

The US Department of Agriculture identifies seven honey colours: water-white, extra-white, white, extra-light amber, light-amber, amber and dark-amber. Certain honeys even have yellow, pink, red, green, blue or even black tones.

A honey's colour depends on its nectar and honeydew sources, the soil and season in which its source plants grew, and its processing and storage.

Plants grown on clay, for example, give rise to darker honeys than those on sandy soils. Autumn, tropical and honeydew honeys are often dark. Heating can darken honey; honey stored at above 0°C/32°F slowly darkens; and honey stored in reused honeycomb darkens by absorbing plant pigments from propolis on the comb. Dark honeys often taste strong because they tend to have relatively more maltose, minerals, acids and antioxidant flavonoids. They also tend to have less glucose and fructose, so taste relatively less sweet.

Spring honeys are usually pale. Light-coloured honeys tend to have relatively more glucose, so crystallize more quickly. They have a mild taste.

Consistency

Honey is runny (uncrystallized) or thick (crystallized) depending on its source plants, processing and age. Most honeys start off runny, but almost all thicken in time, some much faster than others. Some honeys have a gel-like consistency, but liquefy if shaken. Worldwide, most consumers prefer thick honey, though most US consumers like runny honey. Runny honeys vary in viscosity, thick honeys in firmness. Viscous honeys tend to crystallize more slowly than runny ones. Slow-to-crystallize honey eventually tends to form large crystals that can have a gritty texture.

Processors can delay crystallization by heating honey, or by straining or filtering it to remove the pollens, dust, air bubbles and fragments of wax, propolis and bee parts that trigger natural crystallization.

The more glucose a honey contains, the more rapid is the formation of glucose-monohydrate crystals. Crystallization frees the water in which glucose was dissolved, making any remaining uncrystallized honey more watery. Crystallization takes a few hours for high-glucose honeys, a few weeks or months for medium-glucose honeys and a few years for low-glucose honeys. Darker honeys and tropical honeys are generally low in glucose. Some low-glucose honeys remain runny almost indefinitely. Some high-glucose honeys even crystallize in the hive. Certain bell-heather honeys, for example, are so thick that the comb must be crushed before the honey can be extracted. Fast-crystallizing honeys form smaller crystals and are therefore smoother in texture.

Crystallization is also influenced by certain other sugars. Sucrose speeds it up, and maltose slows it down. Melezitose hardens certain honeydew honeys so much that they can't be removed from a hive's honey-box frames; they are called 'cement honey'.

Creamed honey

Processors sometimes induce crystallization by 'creaming'. This thickens runny honey yet prevents coarse crystallization. High-glucose honeys such as clover, leatherwood and sunflower that naturally thicken quickly are ideal for creaming.

First, processors pasteurize the honey to prevent fermentation. Next they 'seed' it by stirring in one part of finely crystallized honey (of the same variety) to nine parts of runny honey. Then they cool it. This triggers very fine crystallization, producing smooth, easy-to-spread creamed honey (also called spun, whipped, candied, granulated, churned or soft-set honey, or honey fondant).

Processors sometimes convert coarsely crystallized honey into smooth honey by heating to liquefy it, then seeding it.

Clarity

Cloudiness in a runny honey generally results from pollens. Frosting around its edge is caused by small air-filled spaces developing during crystallization. Cloudiness can also come from suspended particles of wax, propolis, bee parts and dust. Thick honey is opaque.

Raw honey

Honey labelled raw should not have been:

- Heated. Because even just using an electrically heated knife to cut wax cappings from honeycomb could affect the honey.

- Filtered. Instead, it's simply strained through a wide stainless-steel mesh. Very clear honey has almost certainly been heated to enable filtering, so isn't truly raw.

- Creamed.

- Irradiated.

Raw honey is gently poured or otherwise mechanically removed from the comb, then left for about a week so that risen debris and bubbles can be skimmed off.

Compared with heated honey, raw honey has higher levels of enzymes and scent and flavour compounds. And there is no risk of any other constituents having been altered by heat.

Raw honey is available from beekeepers, farmers' markets and gourmet or organic food stores.

Organic honey

Certified organic honey is free from pesticides and antibiotics. Regulations vary from country to country, but European Union certification, for example, requires the following:

- The hive is kept on land certified as organic.

- Land within 3km of the hive is uncultivated or cultivated organically.

- The land on which the hives are kept is unaffected by significant pollution.

- The hive is made from natural untreated timber.

- The hive has been managed organically for 12 months or more.

- The wax is organic.

- Feeding of bees is with organic honey or sugar, and only between the last honey harvest and 15 days before the first nectar flow.

- Priority for disease control is to build health and vitality through positive management. Unrestricted use of herbal treatments and natural acids (lactic, formic, oxalic) is allowed. After using a prescribed medication such as an antibiotic, the wax must be replaced, and organic status is withdrawn for a year.

Monofloral, blended and honeydew honeys

Blended honeys are the main offerings. Mixed floral (multifloral or polyfloral) honeys are also widely available. But there is growing interest in monofloral (varietal or unifloral) honeys.

Monofloral honey

This has a major input from the nectar of only one particular plant species. This plant may grow in profusion (for example, a crop such as oilseed rape, or the major local tree or wild flower, such as lime, or ling-heather). Or it may be a prolific nectar producer with easily accessible nectar (such as clover or *Asclepias* milkweed). Beekeepers note the flowers their bees visit. If most are of one species, the honey harvested within a day or two of the nectar flow ceasing will be a monofloral honey.

Honeys are sometimes labelled with the name of a particular flower if that species supplies 45 per cent or more of the nectar sources: for example, chestnut nectar forms 85 per cent of most chestnut honey. A higher percentage is extremely unusual, because although bees exhibit flower fidelity, they are rarely entirely faithful! Also, they need a variety of nectars and pollens for good health.

Some monofloral honeys contain less than 45 per cent of one type of nectar. For example, sunflower honey often contains 40 per cent, alfalfa and rosemary 30, linden 25, and acacia, lavender, ling-heather and sage only 20.

Wild flowers account for few monofloral honeys as they are usually so scattered. Exceptions include milkweed, purple loosestrife, rosebay willowherb (fireweed), sainfoin, smartweed, star thistle and wild carrot, all of which are sometimes available as monofloral honeys.

Mixed floral honey

Most honeys are made from the nectars and honeydews from many plant species, with no one being predominant. Examples include summer, autumn, jungle and rainforest honeys, and wildflower honeys. Clover honey's flavour lends such a characteristic stamp to a multifloral honey that this is sometimes sold as 'clover honey'.

Blended honey

Blending different honeys, sometimes from different countries, can lighten the colour, reduce unwanted bitterness (for example, from almond honey) and, if one constituent honey is prone to early crystallization, keep it runny.

Honeydew honey

Any honey can contain some honeydew, but 'honeydew honey' contains more. It's sometimes sold as 'forest' or 'tree' honey. Summer and autumn honeys are the most likely to contain honeydew. Honeydew honey tends to be dark, with strong fig, aniseed or woody flavour notes, depending on its sources.

Tree sources of honeydew include beech, cedar, chestnut, citrus, fir, hickory, juniper, larch, lime, maple, oak, pine, poplar, spruce and willow. Pine and other evergreens are the main source in Europe, beeches in New Zealand. Pine, larch or beech honey is often rich in honeydew. Honeydew honey from fir, larch, linden, oak and spruce trees is rich in melezitose, so hardens fast.

Plant sources of honeydew include alfalfa, beans, clover and wheat.

Characteristics of monofloral honeys

The following table's 'texture' column lists a newly harvested honey's texture. However, most honeys eventually thicken, and any can be creamed.

My favourite is wild carrot honey, produced in Sicily. Others I particularly enjoy are bell heather, buckwheat, clover, ivy, leatherwood, orange, rosemary, tawari and thyme.

Many people pick out apple, black locust, blackberry, milkweed, purple loosestrife, rosebay willowherb, sage and star thistle as being especially good. Everyone has his or her own favourites.

Characteristics of monofloral honeys

	COLOUR	TEXTURE	FLAVOUR NOTES	OTHER
Acacia (wattle, mimosa)	Whitish to pale gold	Runny, unlikely to thicken	Mild, rich, very sweet; floral, vanilla	From Europe, New Zealand, Russia and the US; Europe's major monofloral honey
Alfalfa (lucerne)	Pale	Thick	Not very sweet; mild, floral, spicy; beeswax note; tangy aftertaste	A major honey in Canada and the US
Almond	Dark amber	Runny	Strong, nutty, bitter	Particularly from the US and Spain but often blended because of bitterness
Apple	Pale amber	Thick	Apple	From the US
Arbutus (strawberry tree; corbezzolo; *Arbutus unedo*)	Gold to mid amber; greenish tones	Thick	Strong; slightly bitter aftertaste	From Sardinia, for example; rare and expensive
Avocado	Dark amber	Runny	Rich, caramel, molasses; floral aftertaste	From California, Chile and Mexico
Black locust (locust, *Robinia pseudoacacia*)	Whitish to yellow-amber	Runny, unlikely to thicken	Very sweet; vanilla, floral; fruity aftertaste	From Eastern Europe
Blackberry, raspberry	Pale to mid amber	Runny	Mild, floral or fruity	Mainly from Canada, Russia and the US

	COLOUR	TEXTURE	FLAVOUR	OTHER
Blueberry, cranberry	Pale to mid amber	Runny	Mild; fruity and molasses aftertaste	From the US and Canada
Borage (starflower)	Straw to amber	Runny	Delicate	A major monofloral honey in the UK; also from New Zealand
Broad bean (fava/field/bell/tic bean)	Medium to dark amber	Runny	Rich flavour	From Iran, Egypt and Ethiopia, for example
Buckwheat	Dark purple-brown	Very thick	Strong, caramel, molasses aftertaste	From Europe, Canada, the US and Russia
Cherry	Medium to orange amber	Runny	Almond flavour	A delicious but rare honey occasionally available in Turkey, the US, Iran, Italy and Spain, for example
Clover	Whitish, pale straw or amber	Very thick	Sweet, caramel, floral, new-mown hay, cinnamon	Most common honey in the world; most popular honey in the US
Cotton	Whitish to pale amber	Thick	Floral	From the US and central Asia; cotton is a major source of honey
Echium	Light amber	Runny	Mild; can be tart	A reliable, long-lasting nectar source that is a major contributor to certain honeys from Australia, North and South Africa, and Europe

	Colour	Consistency	Flavour	Notes
Eucalyptus Blue gum (fever tree) Red box gum Yellow box gum	Pale green to gold to mid-amber Dark amber Pale	Thick Very thick Runny	Mild, sweet, herbal, mint; fruity and caramel aftertaste Strong Delicate, fresh, floral	Major honey in Australia and Brazil; also from Spain From Australia Very popular
Fynbos	Amber	Runny	Strong, spicy	From South Africa
Gallberry	Golden to dark amber	Runny	Floral; aromatic aftertaste	Popular in the southern US
Goldenrod	Golden to dark amber	Thick and very smooth	Rich, strong, slightly bitter	From the US
Hawthorn	Pale to dark amber	Runny	Almondy, fruity; slightly bitter; fresh tingly aftertaste	From the UK, France and the US; high in pollen
Heather – bell (*Erica cinerea*)	Reddish-orange to dark amber to ruby	Thick	Strong, woody, minty, slightly bitter	Nicknamed 'The king of honeys'; from Turkey, Scotland and many other European countries
Heather – ling (*Calluna vulgaris*)	Reddish or amber	Thick, jelly-like	Slightly bitter, woody, floral, fruity	Popular in Europe where it's a major monofloral honey
Honeydew	Dark amber	Runny	Sweet, strong, slightly bitter	Contains no pollen; from Europe and parts of Asia

	COLOUR	TEXTURE	FLAVOUR NOTES	OTHER
Ivy	Very pale or straw	Thick	Slightly bitter	From Europe, North Africa and Southern Asia; not usually listed as the main source
Jellybush (lemon-scented teatree, *Leptospermum polygalifolium*; myrtle family)	Dark amber	Thick, jelly-like	Strong, rich	From Australia
Lavender	Golden	Thick	Delicate, sweet, floral, aromatic, slightly medicinal	From France
Leatherwood (*Eucryphia lucida*)	Pale gold	Thick	Strong, floral (elderflower note), spicy; distinctive aftertaste	From Tasmania; organic
Lime (linden, basswood, *Tilia*)	Pale straw or amber; greenish	Runny	Strong, aromatic, floral, woody; lingering aftertaste	From the Czech Republic and Serbia
Macadamia	Amber	Runny	Floral, nutty	From Hawaii
Manuka (teatree, *Leptospermum scoparium*; myrtle family)	Amber	Thick, may be jelly-like	Rich, floral, woody; tannin note; perhaps bitter	From New Zealand
Mesquite	Mid to dark amber	Thick	Sweet, citrussy, smoky	From Mexico, the US and South America

Milkweed (*Asclepias spp*)	Whitish to pale straw	Runny	Mild; slight tang	From Hungary and the US
Neem (margosa)	Mid amber	Runny	Bitter	From India
Oilseed rape (canola)	Whitish to pale amber	Thickens very fast	Mild, peppery	A major honey in Canada, China, Malaysia, Thailand and Vietnam
Orange and other citrus	Medium to dark amber	Runny	Floral, citrussy	Very popular; a major honey in Brazil
Pine	Dark	Runny	Not very sweet; strong; piney; slightly bitter	From Greece, for example
Polygonum species such as smartweed and Japanese knotgrass (Japanese bamboo)	Reddish to dark brown	Runny	Mild	Good late-summer honey in the US; Japanese knotgrass produces dark 'chocolate' or 'blood' honey
Purple loosestrife	Greenish to reddish amber	Runny	Mild	From Europe, Africa, Asia and Australia; not usually listed as the main source
Rewarewa tree	Shades of amber	Runny or thick	Toffee, malt, medicinal flavour	From New Zealand
Rosebay willowherb (fireweed)	Whitish or pale straw	Runny	Very sweet; delicate; tea note	Very popular in the US and Canada
Rosemary	Very pale to reddish-gold	Thick	Fresh, aromatic	From Spain

	COLOUR	TEXTURE	FLAVOUR NOTES	OTHER
Safflower	Medium to dark amber	Runny	Rich, cinnamon, floral	From the US, Mexico and India
Sage	Whitish to bright amber	Doesn't thicken	Mild, herbal	A major honey in the western US
Sainfoin	Pale yellow	Runny	Mild, delicate, aromatic, fruity	This leguminous wildflower and fodder crop grows in Europe, Central Asia and the US; not usually listed as the main source
Saw palmetto	Yellowish brown	Runny	Mild	From the US; not usually listed as the main source
Sidr (jujube)	Dark amber	Runny	Mild	From the Yemen and Saudi Arabia
Sourwood	Whitish to pale amber	Runny	Rich, aromatic, caramel, aniseed, slightly bitter; pleasant aftertaste	From the US
Star thistle	Greenish to pale amber	Thick	Mild; honeysuckle, clover and cinnamon notes	Very popular in the US
Sunflower	Yellowish-white to mid amber	Thickens quickly	Delicate, not very sweet; citrussy	A major honey in Russia

Type	Colour	Consistency	Flavour	Origin/Notes
Sweet chestnut	Dark yellow-brown	Runny, thickens only very slowly	Not very sweet; herbal, toasty; slightly bitter aftertaste	Mainly from France and Italy
Tawari	Golden amber	Thick	Orange blossom; fresh and buttery notes	From New Zealand
Thyme	Golden to reddish to dark amber	Runny	Strong, not very sweet, aromatic; caramel aftertaste	From Greece and the US
Tulip tree (tulip poplar)	Dark reddish amber	Runny	Fairly strong	A major honey in the eastern US
Tupelo (sour gum)	Whitish to pale amber to greenish yellow	Doesn't thicken	Mild, very sweet, floral, herbal, cinnamon, burnt-sugar; fruity aftertaste	Very popular; tupelos grow in the Florida swamplands
Ulmo (*Eucryphia cordifolia*)	Amber	Thick	Aniseed, cloves, jasmine, vanilla, tea, caramel	From the Chilean rain forest
Vetch	Whitish	Runny	Fairly strong	A common source in many countries but not listed as a main source
Wild carrot (Queen Anne's lace)	Deep gold	Very thick	Rich, butterscotch	From Sicily
Wild rose	Mid to dark amber	Runny	Floral	From Greece

What are you buying?

Most honey sold in the UK and US comes from elsewhere, with China and South America the frontrunners. Much is heat-treated and blended. Cheap runny honeys are the most likely to have been pasteurized.

Labelling regulations vary. Ideally, a label should record a honey's weight, whether it has been heated, whether it's monofloral or blended, the country of origin, and where it was packed. A best-before date and the producer's name and address may be given. Any added ingredients should be listed, with their percentages. Sometimes packers add flavourings, for example.

European Union officials are even debating whether pollen – a natural part of honey – should be listed. This sounds odd, given that pollen is a natural ingredient of honey. But it might be sensible as a few people are allergic to pollen, but could consume honey that has been filtered enough to make it pollen-free. Recently, a beekeeper who found genetically modified (GM) pollen in his honey successfully sued the State of Bavaria, which owned trial crops of GM corn (maize). So now levels higher than 0.9 per cent of GM pollen in a honey sold in the EU must be listed, too. As no health risks have been shown from GM pollen, this decision may be to placate the anti-GM lobby.

Occasionally, consumers are misled. For example, while the labels of certain honeys suggest that they are from the home country, they may have been imported (sometimes via a circuitous route to avoid import tariffs or reduce suspicion of adulteration), then just packed in the home country. Also, a '100 per cent pure' label might mean only that the product contains some pure honey. The runnier a honey, and the faster its bubbles rise when the jar is turned upside-down, the more likely it is to contain added sugar syrup.

Finally, some honeys claiming to be monofloral contain only very little of that particular honey.

Aim to buy from trustworthy suppliers: for example, from beekeepers at farmers' markets or from reputable stores.

What to choose

It's worth trying different honeys, noting that:

- Sweeter honeys, which are relatively richer in fructose, go well with cheese.

- When cooking with honey, some of its flavour ingredients will be lost, so you might as well use a cheaper one.

- Mild honeys are better for delicately flavoured dishes and for seafood.

- Strongly flavoured honeys are good on bread, scones or pancakes, on vanilla ice cream, with savoury sauces and meats.

- Acacia honey is good for sweetening drinks without giving a pronounced honey flavour.

- Floral or nutty flavoured honeys suit many desserts.

Storing honey

Bright light destroys glucose oxidase, the honey enzyme that enables hydrogen-peroxide production. So keep honey in a dark place, or in an opaque or dark glass jar, to preserve its antimicrobial power.

Store honey at a cool room temperature.

Honey stored in the refrigerator thickens. If borage honey is refrigerated, it develops a chewy texture like toffee. Most runny honeys crystallize fastest at 14ºC/57ºF. Freezing honey prevents changes in its composition, and the process of freezing runny honey prevents natural crystallization.

Honey stored at warm room temperature may darken and taste stronger because its acidity and enzymes cause a:

- 13 per cent decrease in glucose

- 5.5 per cent decrease in fructose

- 68 per cent increase in maltose

- Slight increase in sucrose

- 13 per cent increase in higher sugars

- 22 per cent increase in unanalysed material.

Because glucose decreases more than fructose, thick honey tends to liquefy when stored at warm room temperature.

Damp air encourages water absorption, which could eventually make honey liquefy or ferment (causing bubbling, cloudiness and an 'off' taste). A plastic container is more air-permeable than a glass or ceramic one. Honey can be stored for years in a glass or glazed ceramic container with a tight lid. Indeed, sealed pots of honey in good condition have been found in 4,000-year-old Egyptian tombs!

In general, properly stored honey keeps well. But storing honey for six months diminishes its antioxidant power by 30 per cent. And storing it for two years begins to reduce its antibacterial power.

Kitchen tips

Keep runny honey in a drip-free syrup dispenser.

If sweetening a hot drink, wait until it's at a drinkable temperature before adding 1–3 teaspoons of honey.

Liquefying thick honey makes it easier to pour and mix. To do this, stand a glass or a microwave-safe ceramic container of honey in hot but not boiling water for 15 minutes and stir occasionally. Or microwave an open glass jar of honey on low for 30 seconds, stir and repeat if necessary. Do this only in a microwave with a turntable, since 'hot spots' could otherwise spoil the honey's flavour. Note that heating honey to 40°C/104°F begins to destroy its enzymes – and the hotter the temperature, the greater the losses.

Honey caramelizes at 70-80°C/160-176°F, with thick honey caramelizing at a lower temperature than runny honey. Caramelization means sucrose is starting to break down into glucose and fructose, producing flavour compounds such as diacetyl (which tastes of butter or butterscotch), hydroxymethylfurfural (which tastes of butter or caramel) and maltol (which tastes slightly burnt).

When measuring honey, coat the spoon or the inside of the measuring bowl or cup with vegetable oil so the honey can slip out easily.

If you would prefer to weigh the honey instead of measuring its volume when using a recipe, note that:

The honey in 1 tablespoonful weighs about 23g/¾oz.

The honey in 1 standard measuring cup (240ml/8 fl oz) weighs about 350g/12oz.

You can substitute honey for sugar in most baking recipes, but:

For each 220g/7oz/1 cup of sugar replaced, use only 165g/5oz/¾ cup of honey, plus one extra tablespoon.

When baking honey-containing cakes and biscuits, reduce the oven temperature by 20°C/25°F as they brown more easily.

Is honey always safe?

Honey can contain potentially toxic substances, or *Clostridium botulinum* spores. It can also trigger pollen or honey allergy in susceptible people. Thankfully, problems are extremely rare.

Potentially toxic honeys

If potentially toxic substances (such as granayotoxin and pyrrolizidine alkaloids, page 30, certain antibiotics, page 35, and certain pesticides, page 36) are present, their amounts are usually too small to be a problem.

Clostridium botulinum

When swallowed into the warm, wet, low-oxygen, low-acid stomach of a baby under one year, *Clostridium botulinum* bacteria spores can germinate and produce botulinum toxin. This can cause botulism within 10 days, with possible symptoms including dizziness, blurred vision and paralysis. One in 100 babies hospitalized with botulism from any food dies.

Honey-consumption is associated with infant botulism in less than one in five cases. Infant botulism is rare indeed in babies of more than six months old. Also, no known case has been attributed to honey in the UK, at least.

Honey often used to be given to older babies. Now, though, to be on the safe side, most experts recommend that babies under one year should not consume honey.

Honey allergy

While rare, there are people who are allergic to pollen proteins or bee proteins and should avoid honey.

Other hive products

These include beeswax, pollen, royal jelly and propolis.

Beeswax

This contains fatty acids, wax esters, hydrocarbons, minerals and carotenoid plant pigments. It is honey-scented, melts at about 60°C/140°F and is available as pellets, granules, blocks or cakes from health food shops and pharmacies (drugstores), or in blocks or starter ('foundation') sheets from beekeepers and craft shops.

Beeswax is present in certain lipsticks, lip balms, body creams, mascara, eye pencils, foundations, shampoos, hair conditioners, dental floss, medical ointments and lubricants, and enteric-coated pills. It's used to make candles, earplugs, crayons and polishes for shoes, floors, skis and surfboards, and is available as a food additive (E901 in the EU; used, for example, as a glazing agent, a clouding agent, a stabilizer and a chewing-gum texturizer). Fruit farmers use it as a graft-wax. And it can even provide a 'green' way of cleaning up oil spills at sea. For this it's made into billions of minute hollow balls that float on the water and allow oil in but not water. Microorganisms attracted from the water to the wax then 'eat' the oil.

Pollens

These colourful, amazingly shaped particles contain the precursors of plant sperms. They are made of proteins (24–60 per cent by weight), amino acids, carbohydrates, fatty oils, lecithin, vitamins (they are especially high in vitamin C), minerals, enzymes and flavonoid plant pigments.

Pollens are commercially available as pollen crumbs or tablets, and in wax cappings. Pollens processed to remove their allergens are sold as tablets.

Some people consume pollen as a health food (for example, to improve fertility, reduce high cholesterol or treat an enlarged prostate, improve circulation or liver function, or to reduce mental or physical stress); as a dietary supplement (for its protein); or to desensitize themselves against pollen allergy. However, the health claims are not sufficiently well proven to be allowed on packaging.

Royal jelly

A hive managed in a particular way can produce just over 450g/1lb of royal jelly a year. This involves collecting royal jelly from queen cells and putting tiny amounts in empty queen cells. Worker bees think these large cells contain queen larvae, so keep them filled with royal jelly.

Royal jelly contains water, proteins, sugars, vitamins (including B5 and C), minerals, hormones, lipids, enzymes, antibacterial substances and acetylcholine. It's commercially available in capsules or phials and used as a dietary supplement and in cosmetics.

It's reputed to strengthen immunity, restore strength, refresh memory, regulate blood sugar, improve the blood count, rejuvenate cells, improve Parkinson's disease and, in children, stimulate growth. But these health claims have insufficient proof so are not permitted on packaging.

Propolis

Certain trees, including pines and poplars, make a resinous sap to deter predators. Bees collect this from buds and bark wounds and mix it with saliva, pollen and beeswax to form a sticky greenish-brown substance called propolis.

This contains resins and gums (50 per cent), waxes and fatty acids (30 per cent), essential oils (10 per cent), pollens (5 per cent) and other compounds (including amino acids, vitamins, flavonoids, bitters and minerals – especially iron and zinc). It smells distinctive, tastes slightly bitter, and has potent antibacterial and antiviral activity.

Propolis is available as capsules, lozenges, tinctures (alcoholic extracts) and creams. It's used in sweets, beauty products and tooth-pastes. It can be mixed with white spirit to make varnish. It's also used for sore throats, asthma, peptic ulcer, gastritis, poor circulation, burns, eczema, warts and piles, and to stimulate new-cell generation. Scientific evidence backs some of these uses.

Baby bees

These bee larvae and pupae are rich in vitamins A and D and protein, marketed in China, for example, as a delicacy and can be deep-fried, smoked, baked or even dipped in chocolate!

CHAPTER FOUR

Natural Remedies

Honey is a popular folk remedy. It's also recommended in traditional healing systems such as Ayurveda and traditional Chinese medicine. Studies convincingly demonstrate that the contents of this amber elixir can be:

- Alkalinizing
- Anti-cancer
- Antimicrobial
- Anti-obesity
- Antioxidant
- Anti-inflammatory
- Capillary (tiny blood vessel) strengthening
- Cholesterol-lowering
- Detoxifying
- Digestion-enhancing
- Immunity-boosting
- Nerve-message-carrying
- Smooth-muscle-relaxing.

The importance of each effect differs from honey to honey.

Honeys originating from medicinal plants may contain some of the compounds in herbal remedies made from their roots, stems, leaves, flowers, seeds or fruits. So perhaps we should think of these honeys as herbal remedies, too.

Choice of sweetener

Refined white table sugar is the most common sweetener in the average westernized diet. High-fructose corn syrup is next and widely used in the US and Japan, though not in Europe. But these sweeteners provide only 'empty calories' because they have no nutritional benefit other than their sugars supplying energy.

Honey, however, not only provides energy, but also contains many health-enhancing compounds.

Honey – an excellent choice

If we choose honey, we tend to consume less than we would sugar, since honey is sweeter and tastes more characterful. Honey behaves differently from sugar in the body, even if we eat a lot of it, because of its acidity, flavonoids and other antioxidants, vitamins, copper and zinc.

Compared with sugar, the average honey makes blood glucose and, therefore, insulin, rise more slowly and climb less high. Certain honeys, including acacia, yellow-box and raw honeys, many high-fructose honeys and runny honeys, make blood glucose rise even less.

This is good, because many health problems (including Alzheimer's, artery disease, diabetes, eye disease, high blood pressure and inflammation) are encouraged by repeated high blood glucose. This encourages oxidation in blood vessels, damage (glycation) to body proteins such as insulin, collagen and certain brain proteins and, eventually, resistance to insulin.

It can help to know about the **glycaemic index** (GI), which ranks foods from 1–100 or more according to their **blood-glucose-raising ability**. (Fats don't raise blood glucose, while proteins do so only in particular circumstances – see below.)

A honey's GI depends on its proportions and amounts of sugars, and on its acids, flavonoids and other contents that influence blood glucose. Choosing a low-GI honey instead of sugar helps prevent unhealthy rises ('spikes') of blood glucose and insulin.

Glycaemic index of honeys, sugars and corn syrups

	GI	FOOD	
Low GI	55 or less	Fructose	19
		Black locust honey	32
		Yellow box honey	35
		Raw honey	30–40
		Acacia, chestnut, heather and linden honeys	49-55
Medium GI	56–69	'Average' honey	58
		Oilseed rape honey	64
		Raw sugar	65
		Sucrose (average of 10 studies)	68
		High-fructose corn syrup – HFCS 42 (42g fructose/100g)	68
		Clover honey	69
High GI	70 or more	Corn syrup	75
		High-fructose corn syrup – HFCS 55 (55g fructose/100g)	87
		Honeydew honey	89
		Glucose	100
		Maltose	105

Bigger liver-glycogen store

Honey is also better than sugar at amassing glycogen in the liver. Glycogen is made from linked glucose molecules, and the liver contains up to 100g/4oz. Liver glycogen is a glucose store and releases glucose to maintain an adequate blood glucose when necessary.

Cells take in blood glucose and burn it as a fuel to produce energy. Brain cells take in 15–20 times as much as other cells yet can store only enough for 30 seconds. They are therefore particularly reliant on blood glucose; they also have first call on it. About a teaspoon of glucose usually circulates in the blood at any one time. Any less and we lose consciousness.

If we go to bed with a low liver-glycogen store, the liver can't top up our blood glucose during the long hours of the night fast. Our cells then need fat or protein as alternative sources of energy.

Fat can be broken down into glycerol and fatty acids, and most cells can burn fatty acids. Fat is an important energy source for these cells, especially at night. While by day most of our energy comes from glucose, during sleep, 70 per cent comes from fat.

But brain cells can't burn fatty acids, because these can't leave the blood vessels in the brain. If low blood glucose continues for two to three days running, the body breaks fatty acids into ketones, which brain cells *can* burn. Until then, brain cells must recruit stress hormones to help get glucose.

Adrenaline, cortisol and metabolic stress

If liver-glycogen stores and blood glucose are low overnight, glucose-depleted brain cells get their energy needs met by recruiting the stress hormones cortisol and adrenaline. These raise blood glucose by making cells resistant to insulin so they take in less blood glucose, making cells burn less glucose and degrading protein so the liver can use it to make glucose.

But stress hormones also raise the blood pressure and heart-rate and make cells burn less fat. And because cells burn less glucose and less fat, they may not have enough energy to work properly.

In other words, stress hormones cause metabolic stress. This can make us sleep badly and have night-time urination, cramp and acid reflux, plus early-morning fatigue, weakness or nausea.

If continued night after night, the resulting chronic metabolic stress can have deleterious effects on health. We risk getting diabetes, artery disease, certain cancers, depression, fatigue, high blood pressure, inflammation, low immunity, memory loss, metabolic syndrome, polycystic ovaries, poor repair of skin, muscles and other tissues, central obesity and osteoporosis.

Honey as a nightcap

Consuming 1–2 teaspoons of a low-GI honey on its own or in a drink within the hour before bedtime is a good way of topping up liver glycogen after a much earlier evening meal and so helping prevent chronic metabolic stress.

Another way is to eat a meal or snack late in the evening, although many people prefer not to eat late.

Which honey to use medicinally

The options include:

- Any honey.

- Raw honey.

- Monofloral honey with particular healing potential; note that certain honeys are allocated a rating for their antibacterial, antioxidant or oligosaccharide activity.

- Honey-containing lozenges, eyedrops, dressings, creams, ointments, gels and patches (from certain pharmacies, drugstores or on the internet).

- Supplements containing concentrated honey extract.

Consume honey as part of a healthy balanced diet, on its own, with food or in coffee, teas or other drinks. Official health advice is to get no more than 6 per cent (in the US) to 10 per cent (in the UK) of energy from sugar, including that in honey.

Honey is generally very safe and often cheaper than other treatments.

Health benefits of monofloral honeys

Honeys vary in their contents and therefore their healing potential. Many folk healers and complementary therapists, including apitherapists who treat ailments with honeybee products, recommend particular honeys.

	Particular health benefits	Uses in folk medicine
Acacia	Antioxidant-rich, fructose-rich	Headache; insomnia; heart, kidney and respiratory diseases
Arbutus	None in particular	Asthma
Avocado	Rich in vitamins and minerals	None in particular
Blueberry	Powerfully antimicrobial	None in particular
Buckwheat	Powerfully antimicrobial; rich in antioxidants (more than 8 times the antioxidant power of clover honey, for example), iron and other minerals, and amylase	High blood pressure; 'rheumatism' and streptococcal throat infections

	Particular health benefits	Uses in folk medicine
Clover	Powerfully antimicrobial; antioxidant-rich; said to increase breast milk	Prevention of heart attacks and strokes; poor appetite; colds, bronchitis; asthma; fever; constipation; high blood pressure; arthritis; burns; kidney disease; anaemia; mastitis; heavy periods; headache; insomnia; tinnitus; neuralgia; epilepsy
Darker honeys	Rich in antioxidants, minerals and, perhaps, vitamins	Infections
Echium	None in particular	Phlegm; brain and nerve disorders, including epilepsy
Eucalyptus	Rich in pinocembrin	Pain; colds, coughs; headaches
Hawthorn	None in particular	High blood pressure; insomnia; artery disease; overactive thyroid; abnormal heartbeat
Heather (bell)	Powerfully antimicrobial; antioxidant-rich; fructose-rich	Digestive problems, cancer
Honeydew	Powerfully antimicrobial; antioxidant-rich; more than twice the antioxidant capacity of honey made only from nectar; rich in oligosaccharides	Sore throat, weakness
Jellybush	Powerfully antimicrobial	Infection, inflamation and wound-healing
Linden	Fructose-rich	Colds; coughs; bronchitis; insomnia; anxiety
Manuka	Powerfully antimicrobial; antioxidant-rich	Infection and wound-healing
Motherwort	None in particular	Heart disease; insomnia; wound healing
Neem	Allergies, diabeties, gum infection, high blood pressure, skin problems, sore throat	Sore throat; high blood pressure; skin conditions; gingivitis; allergy

	Particular health benefits	Uses in folk medicine
Pine	Powerfully antimicrobial	
Raspberry	None in particular	Upper respiratory disease; inflamed mouth; gastroenteritis
Red box gum	Antioxidant-rich	Pain, colds coughs, headaches
Rewarewa	Powerfully antimicrobial	Infections
Rosebay willowherb (fireweed)	Antioxidant-rich	Throat infection; constipation; gastritis; peptic ulcer; skin disease; headache; insomnia
Rosemary	Powerfully antimicrobial	None in particular
Sage	Powerfully antimicrobial; antioxidant-rich	Cough; weakness; kidney and heart disease
Sainfoin	Rich in vitamins (especially vitamin C and beta carotene)	Upper respiratory infection; headache; heavy periods; impotence
Sidr	Powerfully antimicrobial	Constipation; peptic ulcer; liver disorders; eye disease
Sunflower	Antioxidant-rich	Catarrh; flu; asthma; colic; malaria; heart disease
Sweet chestnut	Powerfully antimicrobial; fructose-rich	Respiratory, gut and kidney disorders; malaria; rheumatism; fluid retention
Thyme	Powerfully Antimicrobial; very antioxidant-rich; the most antioxidant thyme honey is rated 10 times as high as clover honey and, weight for weight, 5 times as high as an apple; fructose-rich	Digestive problems, wound infections
Tupelo	Antioxidant-rich; fructose-rich	None in particular
Ulmo	Powerfully antimicrobial; antioxidant-rich (10+)	None in particular

Adverse effects

These are rare, but:

- Many experts advise against honey for under-ones (see page 56).

- Honey stings broken skin slightly in 1 in 20 people.

- A very few people are allergic to pollen, or bee proteins, in honey. Urgent medical help is needed for itching or swelling of the lips, swelling in the mouth or throat, breathing difficulty or faintness after consuming honey.

- People with diabetes or pre-diabetes would probably be wise to avoid the regular use of manuka or jellybush honey with a UMF or ULF of 10 or more (see page 26).

Ailments and remedies

To learn more about a study mentioned here, enter keywords into an internet search engine, plus the journal's name and year.

The suggestions here should not replace any necessary medical diagnosis and therapy.

Acne

Honey kills acne bacteria. Its high sugar content draws pus from acne spots, and its anti-inflammatories soothe the skin.

Action: Apply honey, or manuka-honey cream, three times a day.

Ageing

A survey in the 1980s of some of the world's oldest people found three in four ate raw, unfiltered honey each day.

If honey can indeed help maximize lifespan, one possible reason is that its antioxidants help prevent heart attacks, strokes and cancer.

Another is that honey can boost glutathione – a powerful antioxidant and detoxifier that slows ageing. To produce this from the amino acid homocysteine, our body requires vitamins B6 and B2, and zinc. These are quite often lacking, but honey can help fill the gap.

Also, raw honey may help because it's an alkali-producing food (see page 22).

Action: Consume one teaspoon of raw honey three times a day.

Alzheimer's disease

People with Alzheimer's are prone to oxidation, inflammation and high levels of homocysteine, an amino acid. They also have low (perhaps only 90 per cent of normal) levels of acetylcholine, a neurotransmitter that aids memory.

Honey discourages oxidation, can lower inflammatory prostaglandins and homocysteine, and contains small amounts of acetylcholine.

High blood glucose can encourage Alzheimer's by damaging ('glycating') brain-cell proteins. Honey triggers lower blood-sugar spikes than sugar.

Action: Eat one teaspoon of raw and, ideally, antioxidant-rich honey three times a day, including a teaspoon within the hour before bedtime.

Anaemia

Honey contains iron (vital for haemoglobin), copper (aids iron absorption) and manganese (helps build haemoglobin). The amounts are small, but nevertheless may help.

When 10 volunteers in Dubai took a daily 1.2g of honey per 1kg bodyweight for 2 weeks, blood tests revealed a 20 per cent increase in iron, a 33 per cent increase in copper and slight increases in haemoglobin and red cells.

Journal of Medicinal Food, 2003

Action: Eat one teaspoon of honey three times a day. Ideally, choose dark honey as it's richer in iron.

Anxiety and depression

Pleasure from honey's fragrance and flavour could boost the production of serotonin, a calming and 'lifting' neurotransmitter. Honey contains tryptophan, which can be converted into serotonin. Because honey is a high-carbohydrate, low-protein food, it also helps tryptophan enter the brain.

Honey is particularly good at boosting liver glycogen. A good liver-glycogen store protects the brain's energy supply, preventing the need for stress hormones to take over (see pages 63–4).

Too much of the amino acid homocysteine in the blood is a risk factor for depression; research suggests honey can help lower it.

Chronic metabolic stress (see page 64) can encourage depression; taking honey before bedtime can help prevent this.

Raw honey may be particularly useful as it's an alkali-producing food (see page 22).

In a study at Waikato University, New Zealand, 45 rats ate a
sugar-free diet or a diet containing sugar or honey. After 1 year,
the honey group were less anxious.

Journal of Food Science, 2008

Action: Eat one teaspoon of raw honey three times a day, including one
within the hour before bedtime.

Artery disease

Atherosclerosis narrows arteries with atheroma, stiffens them with
inflammation-induced scarring and calcium deposits, and encourages
poor circulation, strokes and heart attacks.

One cause is high LDL-cholesterol (as this is inflammatory if
oxidized) and low HDL-cholesterol (the protective sort of cholesterol).
Others include pre-diabetes, high blood pressure, blood fats, or homocysteine, and an abnormal tendency to inflammation or blood clotting.

High blood glucose can encourage artery disease by damaging
('glycating') collagen in artery walls and making it less pliable. Honey
triggers lower blood-sugar spikes than sugar.

A test-tube study shows honey discourages blood clotting. The
researchers say this could result from its hydrogen peroxide,
antioxidants, or sugars.

Pakistan Journal of Pharmaceutical Sciences, 2011

In a study of 55 volunteers at Mashhad University of Medical
Science, Iran, the 38 who included 70g of honey in their daily diet
for 4 weeks had lower fasting levels of LDL-cholesterol, triglycerides
and C-reactive protein (a marker of inflammation) than those who
had 70g of sucrose.

Scientific World Journal, 2008

Researchers at Qassim University, Saudi Arabia, found that giving honey to rats helped normalize high homocysteine.

Vascular Disease Prevention, 2006

Also, honey's flavonoids and other antioxidants help protect collagen. This helps keep arteries pliable and strengthens capillary walls, encouraging good blood flow.

Chronic metabolic stress (see page 64) can encourage artery disease by triggering pre-diabetes and high blood fats.

Raw honey may help as it's an alkali-producing food (see page 22).

Action: Eat one teaspoon of raw honey three times a day, including a teaspoon within the hour before bedtime. Antioxidant-rich honey might be especially useful.

Arthritis

Honey contains anti-inflammatories. Honey before bedtime can discourage inflammation (see page 87). Honey's flavonoids and other antioxidants help protect collagen in joints. And honey can lower raised homocysteine, which can be linked with rheumatoid arthritis.

Raw honey may be particularly helpful as it's an alkali-producing food (see page 22).

Action: Eat one teaspoon of raw honey three times a day, including a teaspoon within the hour before bedtime.

Massage honey into the skin over a painful joint.

Bedwetting

Honey is reputed to help prevent childhood bedwetting.

Action: Give one teaspoon of honey within the hour before bedtime.

Burns

Studies suggest honey reduces pain, discourages blistering and infection and speeds skin-cell regeneration of superficial and partial-thickness burns.

Researchers in Maharashtra, India, used honey or silver-sulfadiazine to treat burns in 100 people. After 1 week, 91 per cent of honey-treated burns were infection-free, compared with 7 per cent of the others. Honey-treated burns healed in 15 days, compared with 17 for the others.

British Journal of Surgery, 2001

Action: Apply a honey dressing (see page 94).

Cancer

Test-tube and animal studies suggest that honey has moderate anti-cancer effects and pronounced anti-cancer-spread effects. The constituents responsible include certain flavonoids and other polyphenols. Research will hopefully reveal similar effects in people.

Studies suggest honey:

- Discourages oxidation and inflammation

- Enhances immunity

- Reduces high homocysteine

- Kills bacteria and viruses

- Deactivates certain enzymes

- Detoxifies cancer-causing agents

- Reduces cancer-cell formation

- Reduces cancer-cell proliferation

- Discourages the new-blood-vessel growth that enables cancer growth.

- Encourages apoptosis (suicide) of cancer cells

- Potentiates the anti-cancer drugs 5-fluorouracil and cyclophosphamide

- Prevents the enzyme aromatase, enabling oestrogen production from androgens (male hormones)

- Discourages adverse effects of certain cancer drugs

- Discourages multi-drug resistance.

For example:

A Malaysian study found tualang honey (a forest honey) induced apoptosis of mouth and bone cancer cells.

BMC Complementary and Alternative Medicine, 2010

Research at Greek and Finnish universities suggests thyme honey reduces the body's oestrogenic activity, so could deter oestrogen-dependent breast, prostate and womb cancers.

Food Chemistry, 2009

Chronic metabolic stress (see page 64) can encourage cancer.

Honey's oligosaccharides aid the growth and activity of probiotic gut bacteria, which may help prevent colon cancer.

Honey can aid wound healing in people on chemotherapy or radiotherapy; reduce mouth soreness from head or neck radiotherapy; destroy *Helicobacter pylori* bacteria (which encourage stomach cancer); help prevent infection and odour in cancer involving skin; and reduce febrile neutropenia (fever, plus a low white-cell count: a serious side effect of chemotherapy).

Raw honey may be particularly helpful as it's an alkali-producing food (see page 22).

Action: Until we know more, consume one teaspoon of raw honey three times a day, including a teaspoon within the hour before bedtime.

Cold sores, genital herpes and shingles

Honey helps by excluding air, thus reducing pain, and providing antiviral and anti-inflammatory agents.

Researchers in Dubai, United Arab Emirates, compared honey with acyclovir cream for 8 volunteers with cold sores and 8 with genital herpes. Honey was up to 43 per cent better at reducing pain from cold sores and helping them heal. A similar benefit was found with genital herpes.

Medical Science Monitor, 2004

Action: Apply raw honey three times a day. Or apply manuka-honey cream.

Colds, sore throat and sinusitis

Honey's soothing, anti-inflammatory and antimicrobial properties may help, as may honey's oligosaccharides, which aid the growth and activity of probiotic gut bacteria.

Action: Consume one to two teaspoons of raw honey three times a day.
Or chew some honeycomb for 15 minutes every few hours.
Also, gargle with one teaspoon of honey in half a glass of warm water.

Constipation

Honey attracts water, making stools softer and easier to pass. Also, its acetylcholine stimulates bowel movement.

Action: Consume one teaspoon of honey three times a day.

Cough

Honey's antimicrobials, anti-inflammatories and antioxidants can help. Honey is said to loosen phlegm. Also, honey is safe, whereas certain cough medications can have adverse effects.

In a study at Penn State College of Medicine, 105 children aged 2–18 with an upper respiratory infection and nighttime cough had buckwheat honey, honey-flavoured dextromethorphan or no treatment 30 minutes before bedtime. Honey had the best results.

Archives of Pediatric Adolescent Medicine, 2007

Action: Take one to two teaspoons of raw honey three times a day.

Cystitis

If honey helps, as reputed, this is probably thanks to its anti-inflammatories and antimicrobials. Raw honey may be particularly useful as it's an alkalinizing food.

Action: Consume one teaspoon of raw honey three times a day.

Diabetes

This results from repeated episodes of high blood sugar and insulin leading first to insulin resistance, then to reduced insulin production.

Insulin resistance encourages fat-storage cells to produce oxidants, which, among other things, encourage diabetes.

The amount of carbohydrate we consume is the most important predictor of diabetes, so it's wise to limit its amount. It's also sensible to choose low-glycaemic-index carbohydrates (ones with a low blood-sugar-raising effect) when possible.

Most honeys raise blood glucose less than sugar does. Most importantly, we tend to use less honey than we would sugar, producing an even smaller rise in blood glucose.

Also, honey's:

- antioxidants have a bigger than predicted effect and may, for example, reduce diabetes-related inflammation in blood vessels. In addition, honey is proven to reduce inflammatory prostaglandins.

- flavonoids aid cell communication. For example, eating honey with a starchy food such as bread slows the release of amylase (the enzyme that converts starch to sugar), making blood glucose lower than after starchy food alone.

- trace elements and other minerals may be useful. For example, chromium, magnesium and manganese and zinc are vital for healthy blood-sugar control; vanadium decreases the need for insulin; and potassium improves insulin-sensitivity.

In a study in Karachi, Pakistan, 26 volunteers consumed 1g per kg bodyweight of honey, artificial-honey-flavoured sugar syrup, or glucose. After 1 hour, blood glucose had increased by 20 per cent in the honey group, 47 per cent in the simulated-honey group, and 52 per cent in the glucose group.

Journal of Food Science, 2009

In a study at Mashhad University of Medical Science, Iran, 55 overweight volunteers ate 70g of honey or sugar daily for 30 days. The honey group had lower fasting-blood-glucose.

Scientific World Journal, 2008

In people with pre-diabetes, blood glucose 60 and 90 minutes after eating honey was lower than after eating sugar.

Journal of Medicinal Food, 2007

Eating honey before bedtime may help by preventing chronic metabolic stress (see page 64).

While high homocysteine (an amino acid) encourages diabetes, honey can reduce it.

Lastly, raw honey may help because it's alkali-producing (see page 22).

Action: Use low-glycaemic-index and preferably raw honey instead of sugar in your diet.

Consume one teaspoon of honey within the hour before bedtime.

Eczema

Anecdotal evidence suggests honey can help. If so, this could be because of its anti-inflammatories.

Action: Apply medical-grade honey cream.

Consume one teaspoon of raw honey three times a day.

Eye problems

Topical honey reputedly helps blepharitis (inflamed eyelid margins), cataracts, conjunctivitis, keratitis (inflamed cornea) and corneal injury. If it does, this is probably thanks to its antimicrobials and anti-inflammatories.

It's also suggested that consuming raw honey can help cataracts because it's an alkali-producing food (see page 22).

High blood glucose can encourage eye diseases such as cataracts and age-related macular degeneration by damaging ('glycating') proteins in the eye. Honey triggers lower blood-sugar spikes than sugar.

Action: With an eye-dropper or straw, put one honey eye-drop into the outer corner of the affected eye three times a day.

To make the drops, mix half a teaspoon of runny honey and one tablespoon of warm water in a small container. Make a fresh mixture each day.

To combat infection, use medical-grade manuka (or jellybush) honey. For other eye inflammation, use antioxidant-rich honey.

To help prevent or treat cataracts and age-related macular degeneration, eat one teaspoon of raw honey three times a day.

Fatigue

Honey boosts energy. Consuming it before bedtime can help prevent early-morning fatigue from overnight metabolic stress (see page 64).

Consuming honey before, during and after aerobic exercise reduces post-exertion fatigue as its carbohydrates, minerals and vitamins aid recovery.

Studies suggest honey reduces cortisol during resistance exercise, which would reduce fatigue.

Honey mixed with water is a good alternative to commercial sports drinks. And honey is a good alternative to commercial sports gels. In a study at the University of Memphis, 39 athletes ate protein, plus sugar, maltodextrin or honey after weight-lifting. Only honey maintained optimal blood-glucose for 2 hours (which would aid muscle recovery, glycogen restoration and energy repletion). Blood tests indicated good muscle recovery.

> Presented at the annual meeting of the National Strength and Conditioning Association, Orlando, 2000

Raw honey may be particularly helpful as it's an alkali-producing food (see page 22).

Action: Consume one teaspoon of honey three times a day, including a teaspoon within the hour before bedtime.

Fibromyalgia

Many experts blame this on low-grade metabolic acidosis depositing acidic ions in muscles and connective tissue.

Raw honey may help as it's an alkali-producing food (see page 22).

Action: Eat one teaspoon of raw honey three times a day.

Fungal infection

Honey is reputed to help clear fungal skin infections and research offers some backing.

A test-tube study at Erciyes University, Turkey, tested the effects of various honeys on yeasts such as *Candida albicans*, *Trichosporon* and certain strains resistant to fluconazole. Honey inhibited their growth, the degree of inhibition depending on the type and concentration of honey and type of yeast. Rhododendron and multifloral honeys had more effect than eucalyptus and orange honeys.

Medical Mycology, 2008

Manuka honey with a UMF of 10–15 is reportedly effective.

Action: Apply raw honey twice a day, covering with a dressing if necessary.

Gastroenteritis

Honey's antimicrobials and anti-inflammatories make it useful for bacterial gastroenteritis. Its simple sugars make it easier to digest if gastroenteritis provokes a lack of the digestive enzymes that break down complex sugars. Its oligosaccharides aid the growth and activity of probiotic gut bacteria, which may also help.

Researchers at the University of Natal, South Africa, treated 36 children with bacterial gastroenteritis. Those given oral rehydration solution containing honey recovered in 58 hours on average; those given oral rehydration solution containing sugar recovered in 93 hours.

British Medical Journal, 1985

Action: Consume two teaspoons of antimicrobial-rich honey three times a day.

If unable to keep food down, drink at least 3l/5¼ pints a day of a honey-containing oral rehydration solution made by mixing:

- 1l/35fl oz/5 cups water (boiled if necessary)
- ¼ teaspoon salt
- ¼ teaspoon bicarbonate of soda (baking soda)
- 2 tablespoons runny honey

Gingivitis and tooth decay

Honey's antimicrobials and anti-inflammatories help prevent gingivitis (inflamed gums). Honey can also reduce tartar deposition. Although certain honeys, like sugar, encourage tooth decay, others inactivate the plaque bacteria responsible for tooth decay. This stops them producing acid from sugar. This, in turn, prevents the production of dextrans, gummy polysaccharides that stick plaque to teeth, and reduces demineralization of tooth enamel.

Honeys rich in methylglyoxal are particularly helpful as they act against biofilms such as plaque.

In a study at the University of Otago, New Zealand, 30 volunteers chewed a piece of manuka-honey-impregnated leather or of sugarless chewing gum, for 10 minutes 3 times a day, after eating, for 21 days. The honey group had highly significant reductions in plaque. While gingivitis was reduced by 48 per cent in the honey group, the others had only a 17 per cent reduction.

Journal of the International Academy of Periodontology, 2004

Action: Rub highly antioxidant honey into inflamed gums three times a day.

Eat one teaspoon of antimicrobial-rich honey three times a day.

Hair loss

Honey reputedly slows hair loss.

Action: Once or twice a week, massage two tablespoons of warmed runny honey into the scalp. Wait 30 minutes, then shampoo.

Hangover

Honey's fructose speeds the liver's breakdown of alcohol. Honey also aids recovery by providing sodium, potassium and vitamin B6.

Action: Consume one tablespoon of honey after drinking alcohol.

Hay fever

Consuming locally produced honey for several months before an individual's hay-fever season reputedly helps. Local pollens in honey are reputedly desensitizing. But one study suggests any honey can help:

In a Finnish study, 44 volunteers with birch-pollen allergy consumed honey with added birch pollen, or regular honey, daily from November, and 17 had no honey. In April and May, those taking either honey had fewer and milder symptoms. Those taking honey with added birch pollen used less medication than the regular-honey group and only half that of the non-honey group.

International Archives of Allergy and Immunology, 2011

Wind-spread pollens are much more likely to provoke hay fever as they are easily inhaled. Pollens collected by bees are larger and stickier, so don't hang in the air.

However, nectar is sticky, so may attract wind-blown pollens. Also, bees mix pollen with anti-inflammatory-containing saliva and nectar, and some of this gets into honey. Honey contains vitamin B5, a natural antihistamine.

This may explain why any honey may discourage hay fever. However, locally produced honey is likely to be better, as it not only contains anti-inflammatory-rich pollens and a natural antihistamine but also local wind-borne pollens.

However, another study questions the efficacy of any honey, so the picture isn't clear.

Researchers at the University of Connecticut worked with 36 volunteers with hay fever. One group took 1 tablespoon a day of locally produced unfiltered, unpasteurized honey. The second took non-local filtered pasteurized honey. The third took corn syrup flavoured with artificial honey. Symptoms were similar in each group.

Annals of Allergy, Asthma and Immunology, 2002

Action: Try consuming one to two teaspoons of locally produced raw multi-floral honey three times a day, starting three months before you expect hay fever.

High blood pressure

Honey's antioxidants discourage artery disease; its acetylcholine dilates blood vessels; and its oligosaccharides may help by aiding the growth and activity of probiotic gut bacteria. Honey also helps prevent stress-hormone release (see page 63–4).

High blood glucose can encourage high blood pressure by damaging ('glycating') collagen in artery walls and thus stiffening the arteries. Honey triggers lower blood-sugar spikes than sugar.

Raw honey may be particularly useful as it's an alkali-producing food (see page 22).

All 4,810 volunteers aged 32–86 had normal blood pressure at the outset of a study at Columbia University, but in 647, blood pressure was high 8–10 years later. It affected 24 per cent of those aged 32–59 who slept 5 or fewer hours a night, but only 12 per cent of those who slept 7–8 hours. Affected people were more likely to be overweight and have diabetes and depression.

Hypertension, 2006

Action: Consume honey, in particular, raw honey, instead of sugar. Have a teaspoon of honey within the hour before bedtime.

High cholesterol

A high level of low-density-lipoprotein (LDL) cholesterol, a lifestyle encouraging oxidation of LDL-cholesterol and, perhaps, a low level of high-density-lipoprotein (HDL) cholesterol raise the risk of artery disease, heart attacks and strokes.

Honey raises HDL-cholesterol. Its vitamin B3 can reduce LDL-cholesterol, and its antioxidants help protect LDL-cholesterol from oxidation.

80 obese and 80 other volunteers took 80g honey a day; equal numbers of obese and normal-weight volunteers did not. After 4 weeks, the honey group had lower total cholesterol and higher HDL-cholesterol. Obese honey-eaters also had lower LDL-cholesterol.

Pakistan Journal of Zoology, 2011

Scientists at the National Research Center Dokki in Egypt found honey highly effective at preventing oxidation of LDL-cholesterol.

Evidence Based Complementary and Alternative Medicine, 2009

Action: Eat one teaspoon three times a day.

Immunity

Honey contains immunity boosters.

When 10 volunteers in Dubai consumed a daily 1.2g of honey per 1kg bodyweight, blood tests revealed a 50 per cent increase in white cells called monocytes and a slight increase in white cells called lymphocytes and eosinophils.

Journal of Medicinal Food, 2003

Action: Substitute honey for sugar in your diet.

Indigestion

Honey is said to discourage indigestion.

Raw honey may be particularly useful as it's an alkali-producing food (see page 22).

Action: Consume honey in place of sugar.

Infection

Honey kills many disease-causing bacteria, viruses and fungi. Honey's antimicrobials help counter wound infections. Its prebiotic sugars and probiotic bacteria help prevent intestinal infections and reduce the severity and length of colds.

Honey's immunity-boosters, anti-inflammatories and antioxidants also help.

Raw honey may be particularly useful as it's an alkali-producing food (see page 22).

A Saudi Arabian team that tested 6 supermarket honeys found all retained antibacterial activity even after refrigeration for 6 months or boiling for 15 minutes.

Medical Sciences, 2000

Action: Eat one to two teaspoons of raw or antimicrobial-rich honey three times a day.

Infertility

Honey reputedly increases fertility. Raw honey may be particularly helpful as it's an alkali-producing food (see page 22).

Action: Eat one teaspoon of honey three times a day.

Inflammation

Inflammation is involved in many diseases.

Honey contains anti-inflammatories. Raw honey reduces certain inflammatory prostaglandins. Honey's oligosaccharides aid the growth and activity of probiotic gut bacteria, which may discourage inflammation. Consuming a little honey before bedtime helps prevent inflammation by discouraging chronic metabolic stress.

Inflammation can be triggered by repeated high blood glucose. This is because high blood glucose encourages oxidation in blood vessels and damage ('glycation') to proteins. Honey triggers lower blood-sugar spikes than sugar.

Raw honey may be especially helpful as it's an alkali-producing food (see page 22).

Eating a daily 70g of natural honey for 30 days reduced the inflammation marker C-reactive protein.

Scientific World Journal, 2008

In a study in Dubai, 12 adults had a blood test before and after a 12-hour fast, then consumed 1.2g per 1kg bodyweight (about 1 tablespoon) of raw honey daily for 15 days before another test. Honey lowered the inflammatory prostaglandins thromboxane B(2), PGE(2) and PGE (2alpha) by 48, 63 and 50 percent respectively.

Journal of Medicinal Food, 2003

Action: Consume raw honey instead of sugar. Consume a teaspoon of honey within the hour before bedtime.

Insomnia

Research increasingly backs honey's reputation for aiding sleep. The proposed reasons include:

- Honey boosts serotonin, partly because sweetness stimulates its production, and partly because its tryptophan is readily converted into serotonin. Serotonin calms brain activity and enables production of the 'sleep hormone' melatonin.

- Honey gives a gentle boost to insulin, which also encourages sleep.

- Consuming honey before bedtime promotes sleep by keeping the brain well fuelled.

- Honey can reduce anxiety.

Action: Have one to three teaspoons of honey within the hour before bedtime.

Irritable bowel

Honey may help because of its prebiotic sugars, probiotic bacteria and anti-inflammatories.

Action: Eat one teaspoon of honey three times a day.

Low sex drive

Honey is reputed to help. Jasmine, marjoram and orchid honeys are especially favoured.

Action: Consume one teaspoon of honey three times a day.

Memory loss

Honey is said to help. If so, this might be because it:

- Contains vitamin B and acetylcholine.

- Promotes the production of melatonin (a hormone that helps record long-term memories). People who have honey before bedtime report increased dream intensity and recall.

- Discourages low blood glucose and therefore the production of cortisol which can diminish short-term memory.

In a study at Waikato University, New Zealand, 45 rats consumed a sugar-free diet or a diet containing sugar or honey. After 1 year, the honey group had better spatial-recognition memory.

Journal of Food Science, 2008

Action: Substitute honey for sugar. Consume a teaspoon of honey within the hour before bedtime.

Metabolic syndrome

Also called pre-diabetes, this encourages diabetes, heart disease and strokes and can be associated with polycystic ovaries. It affects up to one in four adults and means having three or more of these factors:

- High fasting blood glucose

- Central obesity

- High blood pressure

- High blood fats

- Low HDL-cholesterol

Eating a low-glycaemic-index honey instead of sugar can help by preventing 'spikes' of blood glucose and insulin and discouraging chronic metabolic stress (see page 64).

Action: Consume low-glycaemic-index honey instead of sugar, including 1 teaspoon within the hour before bedtime.

Mouth ulcers

Honey reputedly helps.

Action: Coat an ulcer with honey every two hours.

Muscle aching and stiffness after exercise

Honey may help because it contains substances that improve glucose uptake and burning in muscles, which reduces lactic-acid production. These include certain acids, flavonoids, glucose-metabolizing principles, minerals and vitamins, as well as hydrogen peroxide and nitric oxide.

Action: Take one teaspoon of honey before, during and after exercise.

Night cramp

Honey's reputed help may stem from its easily digested sugars, minerals or circulation-boosting effects.

Chronic metabolic stress (see page 64) can encourage night cramp.

Action: Take one to three teaspoons of honey before retiring to bed.

Obesity

It's a good idea to substitute honey for some or all of the sugar in your diet. This is because honey is sweeter and more characterful than sugar, so we use less.

During sleep most cells burn more fat than glucose. But chronic metabolic stress (see page 64) reduces night-time fat-burning. It also discourages sleep, thus reducing the 'sleep' hormone melatonin that encourages fat-burning. And it encourages blood glucose and blood fats to be laid down as fat around the waist. Honey before bedtime helps prevent metabolic stress, optimizing the burning of fat to provide energy at night.

Raw honey may be particularly useful as it's an alkali-producing food (see page 22).

In a study at Waikato University, New Zealand, 45 rats were fed a sugar-free diet or a sugar- or honey-containing diet. After 1 year, the honey group had gained less weight.

Journal of Food Science, 2008

In a study at the Mashhad University of Medical Science, Iran, volunteers who consumed 70g of honey daily for 4 weeks had a 1.3 per cent weight reduction compared with those who consumed sucrose.

Scientific World Journal, 2008

Action: Substitute honey for some or all of the added sugar in your diet. Consume one teaspoon of honey within the hour before bedtime.

Pain

Anecdotal reports suggest honey eases pain. If so, it may be because:

- Its sweetness encourages the pituitary gland to release soothing morphine-like endorphins.

- Its sweetness stimulates production of the nerve-message carrier serotonin, which can reduce pain.

- It contains tryptophan and also aids the passage of tryptophan into the brain for conversion into serotonin.

- Its acidity discourages pain related to low-grade metabolic acidosis (see page 22) or high homocysteine.

- Certain honeys contain quinoline alkaloids thought to have a pain-relieving effect.

- Raw honey is alkali-producing (see page 22).

Action: Consume one teaspoon of raw honey three times a day.
Massage honey into the skin over painful muscles and joints.

Peptic ulcer

Methylglyoxal in medical-grade manuka honey kills the *Helicobacter pylori* bacteria responsible for most peptic ulcers.

Helicobacter pylori is 5–10 times more sensitive to manuka than other honey; a 5 per cent solution completely inhibits its growth.
Journal of the Royal Society of Medicine, 1994

Action: Consume two teaspoons of manuka or jellybush honey, UMF or ULF 20, two to three times daily for several weeks.

Psoriasis

Anecdotal evidence suggests honey can help. If so, this could be because of its anti-inflammatories.

Action: Include honey in your daily diet.

Add two tablespoons of raw honey to bathwater, then soak in the honeyed water for 30 minutes.

Apply medical-grade honey cream three times a day.

Skin wounds and infections

People have anointed these with honey since ancient times. Honey:

- Provides a physical barrier against infection.

- Attracts water, which flushes out dirt; prevents waterlogging of tissue; activates hydrogen-peroxide release; draws out pus; enables moist wound healing; and discourages thick scarring (keloid).

- Contains antimicrobials.

- Contains anti-inflammatories that reduce swelling. This reduces pressure on tiny blood vessels, increasing the blood flow and thus increasing the cells' oxygen and nutrient supply.

- Stimulates skin-cell multiplication and gives new cells energy to migrate across the wound.

- Reduces odour within 24 hours, thanks to any remaining bacteria feeding on its glucose. Bacteria in non-honey-treated wounds create foul smells by feeding on amino acids.

- Prevents blood and wound secretions adhering to dressings, so these can be changed without damage and pain.

- Digests dead cells.

Yemeni researchers treated 50 women with a wound infection after a Caesar or a hysterectomy with raw honey or an antiseptic twice daily. The honey-treated ones were infection-free sooner (6 days on average, compared with 15), needed antibiotics for less time (7 days instead of 15) and had faster wound healing (11 days instead of 22). The average scar was only 3mm long instead of 7. None of the 26 in the honey group needed re-stitching, compared with 4 of the 24 in the other group. Their average hospital stay was 9 days instead of 20.

European Journal of Medical Research, 1999

Action: Apply a homemade honey dressing. Any honey helps, but certain honeys are preferable: for infected skin, use raw honey or, even better, medical-grade manuka or jellybush honey with a UMF or ULF of 10–15 or more; for inflamed skin, choose antioxidant-rich honey.

To dress skin:

1. Select a sterile cotton dressing. It need not be non-adherent as honey helps prevent the dressing sticking.

2. Put honey on one side of the dressing.

3. Apply honey-side down.

4. Secure with tape.

5. A larger wound should have a secondary dressing – ideally, an occlusive one (meaning its wound-side surface is made of plastic film, hydrogel or hydrocolloid to prevent it absorbing honey).

6. Change the dressing at least once daily.

7. Or use a commercially produced honey dressing.

CHAPTER FIVE

Beauty Aid

Honey helps cleanse, soften, moisturize, soothe and tone skin and condition hair and nails. Honey's moisturizing power results partly from it helping prevent evaporation of water from the skin; partly from it being a humectant (attracting water from the air); and partly from its acidity (see below). The humectant effect also tones puffy skin by drawing out water. Honey on dry skin stimulates skin-oil or sebum production. Honey's flavonoids improve 'broken veins' (dilated capillaries). Honey helps heal cracked or sore skin and has antimicrobial powers. Its antioxidants reduce damage from polluted air and encourage healthy skin-cell turnover. Honey also enables face-mask ingredients such as oil, ground nuts, egg yolk or clay to stick to the skin. Its fragrance can lift the spirits. Last but not least, honey's acidity maintains or restores the skin's natural acidity.

Skin acidity

Healthy skin has a slightly acidic surface called the acid mantle or hydro-lipid film. This contains fatty acids from skin oil, lactic and amino acids from sweat, and amino acids and pyrrolidine carboxylic acid from dead skin cells. In women, the normal skin pH (an indicator of acidity or alkalinity) over most of the body is 4.5–5.75 (below 7 being acidic, above 7 alkaline). Men's skin is slightly more acidic. This acidity helps repair damaged skin. It also activates enzymes that promote the production of the skin-oil lipids that discourage evaporation of water from the skin (other than from sweat) and deter the entry of harmful substances and microorganisms. The acidity also helps prevent infection by encouraging healthy populations of the microorganisms naturally present on the skin.

Any reduction in acidity – for example, from soap or dermatitis – encourages drying, cracking and itching. Most soaps (even mild, glycerine or baby soaps) and beauty bars have an alkaline pH of 7–9, which temporarily destroys normal skin acidity. This generally recovers between 30 minutes and two hours or more afterwards, although this recovery may be compromised by washing with soap twice daily. Certain soaps are particularly alkaline (pH 9.5–11), and only a very few have the pH of normal skin. However, many liquid soaps, non-soap cleansers and bath and shower gels have a pH that resembles that of normal skin more closely; and a few have the pH of normal skin.

Honey's moisturizing effect results partly from it maintaining or restoring skin acidity, as this helps prevent water loss. A honey-containing cleanser helps retain the skin's natural acidity.

The moisturizing and softening properties of honey's acidity make honey an excellent aid for a manicure or pedicure.

Diluted honey can also restore acidity to freshly washed hair. Most shampoos are alkaline and therefore temporarily destroy the scalp's normal acidity, leaving it prone to dryness, irritation and even infection. Their residues can also make hair look dull. Rinsing with a dilute solution of honey in water makes hair shine. It also makes it more elastic and, in turn, stronger.

When using honey in beauty products, it's often easier to use runny honey. If you use raw honey, you get the added benefit of extra fragrance because it contains the maximum levels of volatile aroma compounds.

Cleanser

- Dissolve 1 teaspoon of runny honey in 4 tablespoons of warm water to make a honey-water cleanser, or

- Dissolve 1 teaspoon of runny honey in 4 tablespoons of warm milk to make cleansing milk.

Gently smooth either of these over your face to loosen grime and dead skin cells. Rinse well with warm or cool water.

Toner

- Use 2 teaspoons of runny or thick honey, or

- Peel and purée 5cm/2in of cucumber, then mix with 1 teaspoon of runny honey.

Apply either of these to your face, leave on for five minutes and rinse off with cold water.

Bath milk

- Use 4 tablespoons of runny honey, or

- Mix 2 tablespoons of runny honey with ½ pint of full-cream milk (or 3 tablespoons of full-cream milk powder).

Stir either of these into a bath of water.

Add extra fragrance by stirring five to six drops of neroli, rose or ylang-ylang essential oil into either mixture.

Moisturizer

- *For normal skin*: mix 1 teaspoon of runny honey with 1 teaspoon of milk.

- *For dry skin*: mix 1 teaspoon of runny honey with 1 teaspoon of full-fat plain bio yoghurt and 1 teaspoon of sweet almond oil.

- *For oily skin*: mix 1 teaspoon of runny honey with 1 teaspoon of extra-virgin olive oil and 1 teaspoon of lemon juice.

- *For ageing skin*: mix 1 teaspoon of runny honey with 1 teaspoon of full-fat plain bio yoghurt, 1 teaspoon of sweet almond oil, the contents of a vitamin E capsule and 1 drop of frankincense essential oil.

Smooth the chosen mixture into your skin. If you make several batches at once, put the mixture into a sterilized jar with a tightly fitting lid and keep it in the fridge for up to two weeks.

You can add extra fragrance to any of the first three recipes by stirring five to six drops of neroli, rose or ylang-ylang essential oil into the moisturizer. The fourth recipe already has extra fragrance from the frankincense oil.

Hand cream

Put 1 tablespoon of beeswax pellets into the upper part of a double boiler and half-fill the bottom pan with water. Bring the water to the boil and simmer until the beeswax melts. Beat in 3 tablespoons of extra-virgin olive oil or almond oil. Remove the bowl and stir in 1 tablespoon of honey, 1 tablespoon of rose water and 1 teaspoon of apple cider vinegar. Cool, stirring, until lukewarm, then stir in 3 drops of essential oil, choosing from chamomile, frankincense, lavender, neroli, rose, sandalwood or ylang-ylang, which add fragrance and encourage skin regeneration. Cool and store in a sterilized jar with a tightly fitting lid for up to two weeks.

Smooth into your hands after washing and drying them. Beeswax pellets are available from health-food stores and pharmacies (drugstores); almond oil from pharmacies; and rose water from pharmacies and certain supermarkets.

Face mask

- *For normal skin*: mix 2 tablespoons of honey with 1 tablespoon of extra-virgin olive oil, an egg yolk and a handful of fine oatmeal.

- *For dry skin*: mix 2 tablespoons of honey with 1 tablespoon of extra virgin olive oil, 2 egg yolks and a mashed banana.

- *For oily skin*: mix 2 tablespoons of honey with 2 whisked egg whites, 1 tablespoon of lemon juice and a handful of fine oatmeal.

Apply any one of these to your face then relax for 30 minutes before rinsing with warm water.

Lip balm

Put 1 tablespoon of beeswax pellets into the upper part of a double boiler and half-fill the bottom pan with water. Bring the water to the boil and simmer until the beeswax melts. Beat in 2 tablespoons of sweet almond oil and 2 drops of an essential oil such as lavender or chamomile. Remove the mixture from the heat, cool slightly, then stir in 1 teaspoon of honey. Store in a small sterilized jar with a tightly fitting lid for up to two weeks.

Apply as necessary.

Exfoliating scrub

- *For normal or oily skin*: mix 1 tablespoon of honey with 2 tablespoons of ground almonds and 1 teaspoon of lemon juice, or

- *For dry skin*: mix 1 tablespoon of honey with 2 tablespoons of coarse sea salt and 1 tablespoon of olive oil.

Rub one of these onto your skin, then rinse with warm water.

Hair conditioner

Mix 2-3 teaspoons of liquid honey into 1½ pints/5 cups of warm rinsing water. To enhance hair colour: *if blonde,* add 1 teaspoon of lemon juice; and *if brunette*, 1 teaspoon of vinegar.

Apply to your hair after shampooing. There is no need to rinse, and the honey will not leave your hair feeling sticky.

Intensive prewash hair conditioner

Mix together 2 tablespoons of honey, 1 tablespoon of coconut oil (from certain supermarkets or pharmacies/drugstores), extra-virgin olive oil or almond oil. As an optional extra, consider adding 1 tablespoon of buttermilk to add moisturizing power and because its lactic acid increases hair strength and elasticity. Wet your hair and massage in the conditioner. Relax for 20 minutes, then wash your hair with a mild shampoo and condition it as usual if you like.

Nail conditioner

Mix 2 teaspoons of thick honey with 2 teaspoons of extra-virgin olive oil and 1 drop of frankincense, lemon or neroli essential oil. Massage this mixture into your cuticles, leave for 20 minutes, then rinse.

CHAPTER SIX

Recipes

Honey's sweetness and flavour enhance many foods, sweet and savoury. And unlike sugar, honey has many health benefits. So it's worth using honey instead of sugar some or all of the time.

Honey helps keep cakes and bread moist and fresh. In a marinade, it tenderizes meat and helps prevent spoiling. Smoothed over roasting chicken or pork towards the end of cooking, it crisps, colours and flavours skin or crackling. It imparts a caramel flavour if the cooking temperature is high enough. And it makes roasted vegetables taste sublime.

Honey is delightful with fruit, porridge, cereals, pancakes, plain yoghurt, cheese and ice cream. It's wonderful on bread, crumpets and scones and excellent in many drinks.

Naturally runny honey, or thick honey heated to make it runny, is usually easier than thick honey to use in cooking.

Please note:

Each recipe serves 4.

1 tsp (teaspoon) = 5ml; 1 tbsp (tablespoon) = 15ml; 1 cup = 240ml/8fl oz.

All fruit and vegetables are medium-sized unless otherwise stated.

All eggs are medium (US large) unless otherwise stated.

If you are using a fan oven, reduce the temperature recommended by 20°C/68°F.

Starters (Appetizers)

Honey's sweetness is a good partner for the sourness and saltiness of goats' cheese and blue cheese. Honey also goes well with the bittersweet earthiness of soups made from root vegetables, and with the *umami* (savoury) flavour of fried sausages.

HONEYED HALLOUMI

Halloumi is a white cheese originating in Cyprus and usually made from goats' or sheep's milk. It firms up when sliced and fried in olive oil, whereas most other cheeses melt. Its saltiness contrasts well with honey's sweetness.

> 350g/12oz halloumi
> 2 tbsp plain (all-purpose) flour
> pinch of black pepper
> 3 tbsp extra-virgin olive oil
> handful of fresh mint or basil leaves
> 2 tbsp runny honey

Dry the halloumi with kitchen paper, then cut it into ¼in (5mm) slices. Put the flour and black pepper into a bowl and stir. Coat the slices of cheese in the seasoned flour.

Heat the olive oil in a large frying pan until hot but not smoking. Add the mint or basil and cook for 1 minute, stirring frequently. Remove the leaves from the pan with a slotted spoon and put them on a plate.

Add the sliced halloumi to the pan and fry for about 1–2 minutes on each side until golden brown. Drizzle with honey and fry for a further 30 seconds. Transfer the cheese to a serving plate, drizzle with any oil left in the pan and sprinkle with the cooked mint or basil. Serve with fresh bread.

BEETROOT SOUP

Honey and lemon juice bring out the flavour of beetroot extraordinarily well. If you buy beetroot ready-cooked (but not in vinegar), you need to simmer the soup for only 15 minutes.

If you use golden beetroot, add ½ tsp turmeric to enhance the soup's golden colour.

50g/2oz/½ stick butter
2 tbsp extra-virgin olive oil
½ tsp ground nutmeg
large pinch of black pepper
1 onion, peeled and sliced
3 sticks celery, chopped
2 cloves garlic, peeled
450g/16oz/2 cups raw beetroot, peeled and cut into chunks
1.1l/40fl oz/5 cups) chicken stock (ideally, home-made by boiling a
chicken carcass – fresh or from a roast chicken – in water with
   vegetables, herbs and spices)
2 tsp lemon juice
2 tbsp dark honey or other runny honey
½ tsp dried parsley, or 1tbsp fresh parsley leaves

Put the butter and olive oil into a large saucepan and heat until the butter melts. Add the nutmeg and black pepper and fry gently for 1 minute. Add the onion and celery and continue cooking for 5 minutes. Add the garlic and cook for another 5 minutes or until the onions and celery are soft but not brown. Add the beetroot and chicken stock. Bring to the boil and simmer for 45 minutes. Stir in the lemon juice and honey.

Pour the mixture into a blender and whizz until smooth. Return to the pan and reheat. Garnish with parsley and serve hot.

HONEY-SOY SAUSAGES

You can use cocktail sausages (each about half the length of a chipolata sausage) or slightly longer chipolatas for this recipe.

    3 tbsp runny honey
    1 tbsp sesame oil
    2 tsp soy sauce
    24 cocktail sausages, cut apart if linked, or 12 chipolatas

Preheat the oven to 220ºC/425ºF/gas 7. Put the honey, sesame oil and soy sauce into a large bowl and stir. Add the sausages and turn them over and over with your hands to coat them thoroughly with the honey mixture.

Put the coated sausages into a large roasting tin. Roast them for 25–30 minutes, or until well browned, turning them after the first 15 minutes. Serve hot or cold on a plate garnished with green salad leaves

Vegetables

Honey adds mellifluous notes to naturally sweet root vegetables. Stir steamed carrots with 1 tbsp butter and 1 tbsp honey, then sprinkle with chopped fresh parsley – simply delicious!

Parsnips roasted in oil and butter are always lovely, but drizzling them with 2 tbsp honey 10 minutes before the end of cooking makes them taste even better. For a change, use a variety of vegetables, as on the opposite page.

THE BEST ROASTED VEGETABLES

Roasting vegetables slightly caramelizes their sugars. Adding honey lends extra sweetness and some caramel notes.

5 tbsp extra-virgin olive oil

large pinch of black pepper

1 tsp ground cumin or cumin seeds

4 parsnips, peeled and quartered lengthways

2 red onions, quartered

2 red or orange peppers, deseeded and quartered

2 green or yellow courgettes (zucchini), unpeeled and cut into 1in/2.5cm chunks

4 tomatoes, carefully scored around their circumference to just pierce their skin

12 garlic cloves, peeled

2 tsp dried rosemary or 2 tbsp fresh rosemary

2 tbsp runny honey

1 tbsp soy sauce

Preheat the oven to 180ºC/350ºF/gas 4. Put the olive oil, black pepper, cumin, parsnips and onions into a large roasting pan. Toss the vegetables in the oil. Roast for 30 minutes. Add the peppers, courgettes, tomatoes and roast for 10 minutes.

Remove from the oven, add the garlic, rosemary, honey and soy sauce turn the vegetables over several times to coat them. Return to the oven and cook for 20 minutes or until all the vegetables are nicely crisped. Serve hot or cold.

RED CABBAGE

Cooking cabbage with very little water helps retain vitamins and flavour. Honey, redcurrant jelly and apple provide sweetness, while apple cider vinegar adds slight acidity. Together, these give delightful sweet-sour notes.

30g/1oz/¼ stick butter
1 onion, chopped
pinch of black pepper
pinch of nutmeg
675g/1½lb red cabbage, trimmed and finely sliced
3 garlic cloves, crushed
4 tbsp apple cider vinegar
240ml/8fl oz/1 cup water
4 tbsp honey
2 tbsp redcurrant jelly
1 large apple, peeled and grated

Put the butter into a large, heavy-based pan and melt over low heat. Add the onion, black pepper and nutmeg and fry gently for 5 minutes, stirring frequently.

Put the cabbage into a colander and wash with cold water.

Add the cabbage, garlic, vinegar and water to the pan and stir. Cover and cook over a low heat for 45 minutes, until the cabbage is tender, stirring occasionally and adding a little extra water if necessary to prevent sticking. Add the honey, redcurrant jelly and apple, stir and cook for a further 15 minutes.

SESAME SQUASH

Honey's flavour goes well with the salty and *umami* flavours of soy sauce, and together they complement the sweet flavour of the squash. Serve sesame squash as a starter or with a main course. Alternatively, insert a cocktail stick into each chunk and serve with drinks before a meal.

1 butternut squash, peeled, deseeded and cut into 1in/2.5cm
   chunks
4 tbsp sesame oil
2 tbsp runny honey
1 tbsp soy sauce
pinch of black pepper
2 tbsp sesame seeds

Line a baking tray with non-stick baking paper. Pre-heat the oven to 180ºC/350ºF/gas 4. Put the squash into a large bowl. Add the sesame oil, honey, soy sauce and black pepper and stir gently but thoroughly. Place the chunks of squash in a single layer on the baking tray. Sprinkle with the sesame seeds and bake for 20–25 minutes. Serve hot or cold.

Dressings and Sauces

Honey is a superb sweetener for dressings and sauces and also adds other flavour notes that depend on its nectar and honeydew sources.

ORIENTAL DIPPING SAUCE

This is particularly good with cooked prawns (shrimp), sliced cooked pork or vegetables. You can make it in advance and store it in the refrigerator for up to 2 weeks. Serve hot or cold.

1 tbsp finely chopped jalapeño pepper

2 spring onions, finely chopped

4 cloves garlic, crushed

3 tbsp fresh ginger root, peeled and finely chopped

3 tbsp coriander (cilantro) leaves and stems, chopped

6 tbsp sesame oil

3 tbsp rice vinegar

3 tbsp soy sauce

2 tbsp runny honey

To prepare the jalapeño pepper, put on washing-up gloves to prevent the pepper irritating your skin. Halve the pepper lengthways and cut off the stalk. Cut out the pith and core, scrape out the seeds and and discard them. Chop the remaining flesh finely. Reserve 1 tbsp for this recipe and store the rest in a tightly covered container in the refrigerator for up to 1 week for use at another time.

Put the 1 tbsp jalapeño pepper and the remaining ingredients into a bowl and stir well.

HONEY-MUSTARD DRESSING

One of my daughters had this honey-mustard dressing on a green salad every day when staying with a French family. She liked it so much that she noted how it was prepared so we could make it at home. Honey-mustard dressing can turn a simple salad or other dish into a meal fit for a celebration. Try it, for example, with goats' cheese and sliced fresh figs.

Using olive and walnut oils instead of olive oil only gives a nutty flavour that is particularly good with hard-boiled eggs.

You can vary the dressing as follows:

- *For beetroot salad*, add 1 tsp of horseradish sauce;

- *For tomato salad*, omit the Dijon mustard and add 1 tbsp of chopped fresh basil leaves;

- *For mushroom salad*, add 1 tbsp of torn fresh coriander (cilantro) leaves.

You can store the dressing in a covered container in the refrigerator for up to 1 week. For a creamier dressing, add 1–2 tbsp of mayonnaise.

    180ml/6fl oz/¾ cup olive oil or half and half olive oil and walnut oil

    1–2 tbsp lemon juice or apple cider vinegar

    1 tbsp Dijon mustard or 1 tsp Dijon mustard and 1 tsp wholegrain mustard

    1 tbsp runny honey

    pinch of black pepper

Put the ingredients into a bowl and whisk well with a fork. Taste the dressing and add more lemon juice (or apple cider vinegar) if you prefer it to be more tart, and more honey if you prefer it more sweet.

BARBECUE SAUCE

Use this piquant sauce to coat beef burgers, pork ribs, chicken pieces or sausages before barbecuing or baking them, or to accompany them after cooking.

3 tbsp tomato purée

2 garlic cloves, crushed

4 tbsp runny honey

2 tbsp extra-virgin olive oil

2 tbsp lemon juice

2 tbsp soy sauce

1 tbsp Dijon mustard

½ tsp cayenne pepper

pinch of black pepper

Put all the ingredients into a saucepan, bring to the boil and simmer gently, stirring, for 3 minutes.

Meat, Poultry and Fish

Honey is a versatile partner for meat, poultry and fish because it adds sweetness and other flavours, and can help brown them and crisp them up.

HONEYED CHICKEN

This sticky chicken dish is bound to become a favourite! If you can't get chicken breasts on the bone, use breast fillets instead.

    60g/2oz/a good ½ stick butter
    2 tbsp honey
    4 garlic cloves, sliced
    4 chicken breasts on the bone and with their skin on
    pinch of black pepper
    1 tbsp fresh parsley

Pre-heat the oven to 180ºC/350ºF/gas 4. Put the butter and honey into a saucepan and heat, stirring, until the butter has melted.

Use a sharp knife to make little cuts through the chicken skin and insert a slice of garlic into each one. Put the chicken into a roasting pan and brush with the butter-honey mixture. Sprinkle with pepper. Roast the chicken in the oven for 40 minutes. Serve garnished with the parsley.

HONEY-GLAZED ROAST HAM

A ham is meat from a pig's hindquarters, cured (in brine or with salt, sugar and spice), possibly smoked, and often called gammon. Bacon, in contrast, is from a pig's side or back. Roast ham is very popular, and honey-glazing it near the end of cooking makes it extra special. Serve hot with mashed potatoes, buttered carrots and cabbage.

Start this recipe the day before you want to serve hot ham, two days before you want to serve cold ham.

Cooking a large piece of gammon means there will be plenty left over to wrap, refrigerate and eat later: cold in sandwiches or with salads; hot and sliced with fried eggs; hot and chopped with pasta or risotto; or in soup.

2.2kg/5lb unsmoked gammon, on the bone

2 bay leaves

12 whole black peppercorns

3 tbsp whole cloves

4 tbsp runny honey

30g/1oz soft dark brown sugar or muscovado sugar

2 tbsp ready-made English mustard

Put the gammon into a large pan, cover with cold water and soak for 12 hours to remove some of its salt.

Remove the gammon, rinse well, then return it to the empty pan and cover it with cold water. Add the bay leaves and peppercorns, bring to the boil and simmer, covered, for 1 hour and 30 minutes. Cool, then drain and pat dry with kitchen paper.

Preheat the oven to 220°C/425°F/gas 7. Line a roasting pan with cooking foil, using a large enough piece so that you will be able to wrap the foil up around the sides of the gammon once you've put it in the pan.

Cut off the rind with a sharp knife, taking care to leave the underlying fat intact. Score the fat into diamonds.

Put the gammon into the foil-lined pan.

Put the honey, sugar and mustard into a small bowl and mix well. Use a palette knife to spread this mixture over the fat on the gammon. Insert a clove into the middle of each diamond. Fold up the foil around any visible meat, leaving the fat exposed. Roast the gammon for 15 minutes, basting frequently and taking care not to let the honey glaze burn. Allow to rest for 10–15 minutes before carving.

LAMB TAGINE

Named after the earthenware pot with a conical lid – *tagine* or *tajine* – traditionally used in Morocco and other North African countries, this is a mildly spiced stew with subtle flavours of honey, orange flower water and cinnamon.

2 tbsp almonds
40g/1½ oz/a good ¼ stick butter
2 tbsp olive oil
½ tsp ground turmeric
1 tsp ground ginger
½ tsp cayenne pepper
large pinch of black pepper
675g/1½lb boned shoulder of lamb, cut into 3cm/1½in chunks
water
2 onions, finely sliced
225g/8oz dried apricots, preferably unsulphurated
4 tbsp honey
4 tbsp orange flower or rose water
1 cinnamon stick
salt to taste

Put the almonds into a large, heavy-based casserole and dry-fry over moderate heat, stirring frequently, until golden brown. Remove and set aside.

Put the butter into the casserole and melt it. Add the oil, turmeric, ginger, cayenne pepper and black pepper and stir. Add the lamb chunks and toss to coat them with the spices and oil. Fry the meat, stirring, for 5 minutes. Add enough water to cover the meat. Bring to the boil, reduce the heat, cover and cook for 1 hour.

Stir in the onion and cook for 30 minutes more. Stir in the apricots, honey and orange flower or rose water and add the cinnamon stick. Check the seasoning, adding salt to taste. With the casserole uncovered, simmer for 5 minutes or until the apricots have plumped up. Remove from the heat, scatter the meat with the almonds and serve hot with couscous or rice.

MARINATED SALMON

Covering fresh filleted salmon in salt and honey, then wrapping and leaving it in a cool dark place for several days, cures or 'cold-cooks' it, producing a delicacy even more special than smoked salmon. Flavourings such as fresh dill provide extra interest.

Another idea that provides interesting colour and flavour is to add grated cooked beetroot (without vinegar).

1 side of salmon weighing about 1kg/2.2 lb, filleted but not
   skinned
300g/11oz/1 cup table salt
240ml/8fl oz/1 cup runny honey
1 handful fresh dill

Line a roasting pan with enough cooking foil to wrap loosely around and cover the salmon.

Run the flats of your fingers over the inside of the salmon fillet to check for any small 'pin' bones. If you find any, remove them with a pair of pliers or strong tweezers. Cut the salmon fillet in half across its length. Lay one piece, skin side down, on the foil in the roasting pan. Sprinkle with salt, drizzle with honey and cover with about half the dill. Lay the other piece of salmon, skin side up, on top of the first one. Wrap the foil loosely over the salmon, put it in the refrigerator and leave for about 36 hours.

Remove from the fridge, pull back the foil, pick up the two pieces of salmon together and turn them upside down. Wrap the foil back over the salmon and put the pan back in the refrigerator for another 36 hours or so.

Unwrap the salmon pieces and wash them under running cold water for 1–2 minutes. Pat them dry with kitchen paper. Put one of the pieces skin side down on a flat surface. Hold one end of it with one hand and with a large sharp knife cut slices from the salmon with the other hand, moving the knife away from you. The slices can be as thick or as thin as you like. Continue until you have removed all the salmon from the skin. The brownish part closest to the skin is the most delicious (and also the most rich in health-giving omega-3 fatty acids). Repeat with the other piece of salmon. Put the slices on a large plate and serve with lemon wedges, brown bread and butter.

Desserts

Honey makes a fine replacement for sugar in desserts as varied as bread and butter pudding; cheesecake; poached, barbecued fruits or baked fruits; and ice creams and sorbets. It's also lovely drizzled over soft cheeses.

FLUMMERY

Also called Atholl Brose, this hails from Scotland. While delicious in its own right, it's also very good with fresh raspberries.

    1 level tbsp oatmeal
    300ml/½ pint/1¼ cups double cream
    3 tbsp whisky
    3 tbsp runny honey
    1 tbsp lemon juice

Toast the oatmeal by dry-frying it in a heavy-based frying pan, stirring occasionally, until it browns. Cool. Put the cream into a bowl and whisk until slightly thickened. Continue to whisk while gradually adding the whisky. Stir in the honey, lemon juice and toasted oatmeal.

APPLES FRIED IN HONEY AND BUTTER

Coxes and Egremont Russets are among the best dessert apples for this dish.

    50g/2oz/½ stick butter
    25g/1oz brown sugar
    zest and juice of 1 large orange

juice of ½ lemon

3 tbsp honey

4 dessert apples

Melt the butter in a frying pan. Add the sugar, orange juice and zest, lemon juice and honey and heat gently, stirring occasionally. Peel, quarter and core the apples, then halve each piece lengthways. Add the apples to the pan and cook gently for 10–15 minutes, turning them over every so often. Serve hot with vanilla ice cream, double cream or crème fraîche.

SEMOLINA WITH HONEY AND DATES

Using honey instead of sugar and adding dates turns semolina from satisfying comfort food into an instant hit.

600ml/1 pint/2½ cups milk

45g/1½oz semolina

2 tbsp honey

15g/½oz butter

75g/3oz chopped dates

Put the milk into a saucepan and heat until lukewarm. Stir in the semolina and heat until the mixture comes to the boil and thickens, stirring frequently. Add the honey, butter and dates and stir well. Cook for a further 5 minutes, stirring frequently to prevent burning.

Cakes, Biscuits and Bread

Honey is an excellent sweetener for baked goods. Apart from the honey cake and other recipes below, honey is particularly successful in banana loaf, muffins and gingerbread.

BAKLAVA

This delightful Greek dessert consists of exceedingly thin sheets of pastry separated by a layer of chopped nuts and soaked with honey syrup. It's also popular in Armenia, Croatia, Cyprus, Macedonia, Serbia, Slovenia and the near and middle East.

FOR THE SYRUP
330ml/11fl oz/1¼ cups warm water
200g/7oz/1 cup sugar
4 cloves
1 cinnamon stick
juice and finely grated zest of 1 orange
240ml/8fl oz/1 cup runny honey
2 tbsp rosewater

FOR THE PASTRY
150g/5oz finely chopped pistachios
150g/5oz finely chopped walnuts
2 tbsp caster sugar
1 tsp ground cardamom
18 ready-made filo-pastry sheets
250g/9oz/2½ sticks butter, melted

Preheat the oven to 180°C/350°F/gas 4. Brush a rectangular baking tin with a little melted butter.

Make the syrup by putting the water, sugar, cloves, cinnamon stick and orange juice and zest into a pan. Heat gently until the sugar has dissolved. Bring to the boil and simmer for 15 minutes. Add the honey and simmer for 2 minutes. Cool, then remove the cinnamon stick and stir in the rosewater.

Reserve 2 tbsp of chopped pistachios. Put the remaining pistachios, walnuts, sugar and cardamom into a bowl and stir.

Lay a pastry sheet in the baking tin, cutting it if necessary so that it fits. Brush with a little melted butter. Repeat until you have used 9 sheets. Spread the nut, sugar and cardamom mixture over the pastry-sheet stack. Add another pastry sheet and brush it with melted butter. Repeat until you have used all the sheets.

With a sharp knife, cut a diamond pattern halfway down into the baklava.

Bake for 20 minutes, then reduce the heat to 150°C/300°F/gas 2 for 35–40 minutes and bake until golden brown. Remove from the oven and cut the diamond-shaped pieces right through. Strain the syrup and pour it over the baklava. Cool, then scatter with the remaining pistachios.

HONEYCAKE

The first honeycakes were made from rye flour and honey. In the Middle Ages, cooks began to add spices. They rested the dough for weeks before baking it so that the honey could ferment and aerate the dough.

Most modern honeycakes contain baking powder or another modern raising agent, plus butter and, perhaps, other refinements such as nuts. Rye flour has largely been superseded by white or wholemeal flour (or both).

240ml/8fl oz/1 cup dark honey or other runny honey
50g/2oz caster sugar
175g/6oz/¾ cup melted butter
2 tsp instant coffee
4 eggs, beaten
150g/5oz/1 ⅓ cups white self-raising flour
150g/5oz/1 ⅓ cups wholemeal self-raising flour
½ tsp ground cinnamon
½ tsp ground cloves
½ tsp ground star anise
120ml/4fl oz/½ cup milk

Preheat the oven to 180ºC/350ºF/gas 4. Line a 25cm/10in diameter cake tin with non-stick baking parchment.

Put the honey, sugar, butter and coffee into a large bowl and beat until well creamed. Beat in the eggs a little at a time. Put the flour, cinnamon, cloves and star anise into another bowl and stir. Sift a little of this into the honey mixture, then stir in a little of the milk. Repeat until you have used all the flour, spices and milk.

Pour the mixture into the cake tin and bake for 40 minutes. Reduce the heat to 170ºC/325ºF/gas 3 and bake for a further 20 minutes or until a skewer stuck into the middle of the cake comes out clean. Let it cool in the tin for 5 minutes, then transfer the honeycake to a wire rack to cool completely.

HONEY SHORTBREAD

This shortbread is so smooth that it simply melts in the mouth.

225g/8oz/2 sticks butter
120ml/4fl oz/½ cup runny honey
1 tsp vanilla extract
250g/9oz/2½ cups plain flour

Preheat the oven to 150ºC/300ºF/gas 2. Lightly grease a non-stick baking tray or line an ordinary baking tray with non-stick baking paper.

Put the butter, honey and vanilla extract into a large bowl and beat until light and fluffy. Gradually add the flour, mixing well with each addition. Turn the dough onto a lightly floured board and flatten evenly but gently to about ½ in (12mm) thick.

Place the flattened dough on the baking tray. Score 24 rectangles into the dough with a sharp knife. Prick all over with a fork. Bake for 35–40 minutes. Cool for 10 minutes, then transfer to a wire rack to cool completely.

RAISIN CHALLAH

Jewish families traditionally eat two loaves of this plaited egg-enriched yeast bread at each of the three meals over Shabbat (the Sabbath). They also eat this bread on ceremonial occasions and during festive holidays. The loaf is formed from six woven strands of dough instead of the three usually braided into a plait. This 'double' loaf commemorates the manna that apparently fell from heaven to help sustain the Israelites during their 40 years of exile in the desert after their exodus from Egypt. And the twelve strands of dough needed to make two loaves remind diners of the twelve tribes of Israel.

The manna mentioned in the Bible was almost certainly honeydew – a sweet, dark or greenish liquid or crystalline substance excreted by aphids, leafhoppers and scale insects on to leaves or branches after eating a tree's sap. It's called honeydew because its droplets glisten like dew.

My version of challah is therefore sweetened with honey to represent manna.

Enjoy it for breakfast or with tea or coffee in the afternoon. It's also delicious slightly toasted and spread with butter and honey or homemade jam.

240ml/8fl oz warm water
2 tsp dried yeast
1 egg, beaten
1 tbsp vegetable oil
175g/6oz raisins (optional)
4 tbsp runny honey
400g/14oz/4 cups plain flour
1 tbsp coarse sea salt

FOR THE GLAZE
1 egg, beaten
2 tbsp poppyseeds or sesame seeds (optional)

Put the water, yeast, egg, oil, optional raisins, and honey into a large bowl. Mix well, add half the flour and mix well again. Leave for 1 hour at warm room temperature.

Add the salt and the remaining flour and mix well. Turn out the dough onto a lightly floured surface and knead until stretchy. Divide it into six pieces and roll each into a long spindle shape. Lay the pieces alongside each other and press one end of each one together. Now plait (braid) the six pieces, then press their remaining free ends together. Put the plait onto an oiled baking sheet and leave to rise for at least 1 hour.

Preheat the oven to 180°C/350°F/gas 4. Glaze the loaf with the beaten egg and sprinkle with the poppyseeds or sesame seeds if you wish. Transfer the baking sheet into the oven and bake for 45 minutes. Remove from the baking sheet and cool on a wire rack.

Useful Websites

Here are some of the organizations concerned with honey and beekeeping around the world.

United Kingdom
British Beekeepers Association
www.bbka.org.uk
Umbrella body for local beekeeping associations
Provides information on bee stings, honeybees and pesticides, and shrubs and trees useful to bees.

UK Honey Association
www.honeyassociation.com
Website of the British Honey Importers and Packers Association
Provides information about honey as well as honey recipes.

National Bee Unit
www.nationalbeeunit.com
A beekeeping-resource website

Royal Horticultural Society
www.rhs.org.uk/Gardening/Sustainable-gardening/pdfs/
RHS_Polinators_PlantList_V1
This takes you to a useful list of plants that attract bees season by season.

United States

National Honey Board

www.honey.com

Represents producers, packers, importers and a marketing cooperative and organizes research, marketing and promotion for honey and honey products.

The website includes information about honey as well as honey recipes. To locate particular honeys in the US, visit the National Honey Board website: http://www.honeylocator.com/locator/home/

American Honey Producers Association

www.americanhoneyproducers.org

An organization for beekeepers that also offers industry news and cooking tips

Certified Naturally Grown

www.naturallygrown.org

An independent organization that offers information on best practices for honey production, and certification to beekeepers who follow this practice. It also gives information on honey.

Australia

Australian Honey Bee Industry Council

www.honeybee.org.au

Represents beekeepers and encourages best practice in production, quality assurance, presentation and promotion of its products.

New Zealand

National Beekeepers Association of New Zealand

www.nba.org.nz

Canada

Canadian Honey Council

www.honeycouncil.ca

Besides offering beekeeping information, this has information about the honey industry.

Index